ART THERAPY
AND PSYCHOTHERAPY

ART THERAPY AND PSYCHOTHERAPY

Blending Two Therapeutic Approaches

Victoria D. Coleman, Ed.D.
Phoebe M. Farris-Dufrene, Ph.D.

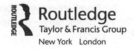
Routledge
Taylor & Francis Group
New York   London

First published by Accelerated Development

This edition published 2013 by Routledge

Routledge
Taylor & Francis Group
711 Third Avenue
New York, NY 10017

Routledge
Taylor & Francis Group
2 Park Square, Milton Park
Abingdon, Oxon OX14 4RN

Routledge is an imprint of the Taylor & Francis Group, an informa business

ART THERAPY AND PSYCHOTHERAPY: Blending Two Therapeutic Approaches

This book was set in Times Roman by Sandra F. Watts. Technical development and editing by Cynthia Long. The pre-press supervisor was Bonny Gaston. Cover design by Michelle Fleitz. Cover photo adapted from Figure 15, "Donald: Flower." Printing and binding by Braun-Brumfield, Inc.

A CIP catalog record for this book is available from the British Library.

Library of Congress Cataloging-in-Publication Data
Coleman, Victoria, D.
  Art therapy and psychotherapy: blending two therapeutic approaches/Victoria D. Coleman, Phoebe M. Farris-Dufrene.
    p. cm.

  1. Art therapy—Case studies.   2. Psychotherapy—Case studies.   I. Title.
  [DNLM: 1. Art Therapy. 2. Psychotherapy—methods. 3. Art Therapy—case studies.   WM 450.5.A8   C692a   1996]
RC489.A7C65   1996
616.89'1656—dc20
DNLM/DLC
for Library of Congress   95-26439
ISBN 1-56032-489-9 (cloth)   CIP
ISBN 1-56032-490-2 (paper)

To my mother, Jacqueline I. Moore

v.d.c.

To my mother, Phoebe Lyles, and my daughter, Sienna Farris

p.f.d.

TABLE OF CONTENTS

LIST OF FIGURES

Preface

Psychotherapy is a state of art of healing used to treat a variety of psychiatric disorders from time immemorial; it became firmly established in the Freudian era, and the term "psychotherapy" was coined. In fact, psychotherapy was the only treatment modality available to psychiatrists and psychotherapists for over a century until the advent of medications and other somatic therapies.

Basically, two kinds of problems brought people to psychiatric providers—those that seem to have their origins largely in the remote past, and those that seem to arise largely from current stresses, both internal and external. Psychoanalysis became the preferred approach in dealing with the former, while a multitude of other therapies evolved to deal with the latter, some of them extremely creative and clever and far less time consuming than the conventional psychoanalytical approach.

Amidst such, Dr. Coleman and Dr. Farris-Dufrene have come up with yet another novel approach to treating psychiatric disorders by combining their expertise of psychotherapy and art therapy, respectively, which I am sure will go a long way in effecting maximal benefits to their clientele and improving and enriching the quality of their lives.

These therapies can be used effectively in conjunction with somato- and psychopharmacotherapies as they complement one another.

In closing, I highly recommend this book to all practicing therapists, as well as students training to become therapists, and would not be surprised if this book is included in school curricula throughout the nation.

Mohammed Q. Fazal, M.D.
Assistant Professor of Psychiatry
Chicago Medical School
Chicago, Illinois

ACKNOWLEDGMENTS

Many individuals have assisted us in the development of this book. As we acknowledge our indebtedness, we regret that we cannot identify all of them.

Foremost, we are grateful to Dr. Joseph Hollis, publisher of Accelerated Development/Taylor & Francis, for his confidence in our abilities as therapists and authors. He was extremely patient and provided exceptional feedback as we deliberated in this scholarly endeavor.

For referring many of our clients, we would like to thank Ms. Andrea McKay of the Charter Behavioral Health System, Lafayette, Indiana. The professional development workshops and networking opportunities provided by Charter were invaluable in our research for this book.

A special thanks to Dr. William C. Bingham, Professor Emeritus, Rutgers University, doctoral advisor and mentor, who helped prepare me (Victoria Coleman) as a counseling psychologist. Also, Dr. Duncan Walton, a member of my dissertation committee, whose insight on multicultural populations helped me immensely in my career.

For his untiring assistance in the development of my dissertation and preparation as a university professor, I (Phoebe Farris-Dufrene) am indebted to Dr. Randall Craig, University of Maryland, College Park. I also would like to give thanks to Mr. Cliff Joseph, ATR, my master's thesis advisor at Pratt Institute.

At Purdue University, we are indebted to Dr. James P. Greenan and Dr. Peter Smith, who provided support and feedback during the various stages of this book. Ms. Marilyn B. Rogers, graduate assistant, conducted the computer search for the review of the literature.

To all of the children, adolescents, adults, and families with whom we have worked throughout the years, you have taught us much more than could ever be discerned from merely reading a book. We have enjoyed our interactions and wish you success in your personal growth and development.

V.D.C.
P.F.D.

Chapter 1

INTRODUCTION

As the world changes rapidly, helping professionals and educators must reevaluate their philosophies, goals, and objectives in order to interact with diverse populations. In the last decade of the twentieth century, our nation is being challenged to develop new conceptualizations, paradigms, definitions, strategies, and techniques for surviving in the intense, competitive, global economy. As these changes impact all individuals, it has become necessary for mental health professionals to expand their knowledge of therapeutic approaches.

Due to the myriad of changes in the mental health profession, the authors recognized the need to fuse various treatment methodologies in order to provide better services to clients. Each of the authors has extensive experience working with clients who have a multitude of disorders ranging from neuroses to psychoses. In addition, the therapists provide services to clients from a variety of socioeconomic, racial, and ethnic backgrounds.

Coming to Purdue University in 1989 to pursue academic careers, the authors also had an opportunity to utilize their clinical skills in the community. Because of mutual interests in therapeutic interventions for multicultural populations, the therapists decided to collaborate on a number of projects, including research and scholarly activities, and serving as cotherapists. In their efforts as cotherapists, they identified trends and patterns of behavior prevalent among the clients that were seen. Some of the problems impacting upon their clients were physical and sexual abuse, racial oppression and discrimination, dysfunctional family systems, and a lack of support from the juvenile/adult judicial system and the state welfare department.

After discussion and analysis of the aforementioned situations, the authors determined the importance of reporting their findings to the mental health profession. Consequently, collaboration on a book seemed an appropriate activity. Because of Coleman's background in psychotherapy, and Farris-Dufrene's expertise in art therapy, it was decided to fuse the two disciplines.

Coleman's educational training and professional experience include positions in higher education, corporate America, mental health services, social services, and entrepreneurship. Her doctoral work in counseling psychology focused on self-concept development, which has its antecedents in the theoretical framework of Super's (1957) Developmental Self-Concept Theory of Vocational Behavior. Super, considered the father of vocational psychology, has suggested that individuals attempt to implement their self-concept by choosing to pursue an occupation that they perceive would provide the most opportunity for self-expression.

Utilizing Super's (1957) framework as the foundation for individual, group, and family counseling, Coleman has focused on the self-concept development of multicultural and diverse populations. Major components of the self-concept are self-esteem, the feeling tone, self-acceptance, and/or how one feels about oneself (Super, Starishevsky, Matlin, & Jordaan, 1963). As many of her clients present with depression and low self-esteem, it is within these constructs that she has focused on their personal growth and development.

While working in a variety of venues, Coleman has been exposed to many individuals, families, and groups that were not particularly receptive to the traditional "talk" psychotherapy. Having collaborated with Farris-Dufrene, an art therapist, on research, publications, and conference presentations, it was natural that the two would work together clinically to accommodate the nonverbal clients.

Farris-Dufrene utilizes both the art as therapy approach and art psychotherapy, depending on the work environment and the client's needs. When she is working in private practice as a primary therapist, cotherapist, or art therapy consultant, she functions more as an art psychotherapist. However, when working in psychiatric or educational institutions that employ other personnel such as psychiatrists, psychiatric nurses, social workers, etc., she prefers the art as therapy approach, leaving the psychotherapy to other mental health professionals.

Farris-Dufrene's approach to dealing with behavioral issues, both during the art therapy sessions and in the client's other domains, is one that attempts to assist in developing the client's ego capacities through the use of reality testing and appraisal in abeyance through self-control and constructive channeling (Henley, 1992). Offering creative outlets for energy discharge increases the client's capacity for sublimation and motivation. It is a behavioral approach that employs sympathy for one's clients without being overly permissive. It implies an acceptance of art that may be violent or overtly sexual, while at the same time encouraging clients to distinguish between creating emotionally charged art and acting out those feelings in a manner that could harm others or themselves (Henley, 1992).

Art therapy and psychotherapy are obviously compatible as witnessed by the collaboration between the two authors in clinical and scholarly endeavors. Each has its purpose with respect to facilitating the personal growth and development of individuals, families, and groups. It is within this context that this book, *Art Therapy and Psychotherapy: Blending Two Therapeutic Approaches*, was conceptualized.

The purpose of this book is to provide an opportunity for mental health professionals to gain "hands on" information related to these two modalities. The mental health profession is in need of specific tools that can help facilitate the counseling process, and the use of different techniques will allow therapists to be more equipped to handle a variety of issues and situations as they assist individuals, families, and groups in seeking self-actualization.

This book utilizes the case study approach in order to provide mental health professionals with specific examples for treatment of various disorders. Cases include art illustrations by children and adults while in therapy, diagnoses, in-depth discussion of the art therapy and psychotherapy sessions, and recommendations.

This book also can serve as a resource for students, university educators, and clinicians. Each chapter of the book is highlighted below.

CHAPTER 1—INTRODUCTION

In this chapter is presented an introduction to issues and concerns faced by mental health professionals as they attempt to blend two therapeutic modalities. It also includes a brief statement of the contents of each chapter.

CHAPTER 2—THEORETICAL FRAMEWORK
AND REVIEW OF THE LITERATURE

The authors present the antecedents of their theoretical frameworks and discuss how pioneers in art therapy and psychotherapy have influenced the blending of two approaches.

CHAPTER 3—BLENDING ART THERAPY
AND PSYCHOTHERAPY

The purpose of this chapter is to present a conceptualization for blending art therapy and psychotherapy. This chapter discusses the interdisciplinary nature of art therapy, which encompasses art, psychology, and therapy. The use of a variety of disciplines makes art therapy conducive to the work of many mental health professionals, particularly psychotherapists.

CHAPTER 4—CASE STUDIES:
CHILDREN AND ADOLESCENTS

In Chapter 4 are highlighted two case studies, one involving three siblings who were victims of sexual abuse, and the other two siblings dealing with issues of adoption. This chapter also outlines the various agencies and organizations that impact upon the treatment of children and adolescents.

CHAPTER 5—CASE STUDIES: FAMILIES

In this chapter are emphasized the complexities of working with a dysfunctional family that had been involved with the juvenile and adult judicial system, as well as the state welfare department. The discussion focuses on treating the entire family.

CHAPTER 6—CASE STUDIES: ADULTS

Two adult females and one adult male are profiled in this chapter. Case Study #1 involves a middle-aged Middle Eastern woman who suffered posttraumatic stress syndrome. The second case highlights career related stress in mid-life. The third case involves an urban Native American dealing with job discrimination and a recent divorce.

CHAPTER 7—PROFESSIONAL, ETHICAL, AND LEGAL CONSIDERATIONS

In Chapter 7 are identified specific professional, ethical, and legal issues that should be considered when providing art therapy and psychotherapeutic services. Some of the topics addressed are codes of ethics, confidentiality, civil and criminal liability, and private practice. Guidelines are formulated on principles established by the American Psychological Association.

CHAPTER 8—MULTICULTURAL ISSUES IN ART THERAPY AND PSYCHOTHERAPY

In Chapter 8, readers are informed of the considerations in working with multicultural and diverse populations. These populations include ethnic minorities, biracial clients, and clients of various socioeconomic levels. The authors suggest the appropriateness of providing clients with the option to select therapists of their own cultural background.

CHAPTER 9—CAREER DEVELOPMENT ISSUES IN ART THERAPY AND PSYCHOTHERAPY

The career development of art therapists and psychotherapists is discussed based on a model designed by one of the authors. The model focuses on self-assessment; decision making; educational, occupational, and community information; and preparation for work, leisure, and retirement.

CHAPTER 10—IMPLICATIONS FOR MENTAL HEALTH PROFESSIONALS

The final chapter of this book is concerned with significant implications related to art therapy, psychotherapy, training, research, program development, and policy. It reinforces that the blending of art therapy and psychotherapy is a feasible orientation for mental health professionals.

REFERENCES

Henley, D. (1992). *Exceptional children: Exceptional art.* Worcester, MA: Davis Publications.

Super, D.E. (1957). *The psychology of careers.* New York: Harper & Row.

Super, D.E., Starishevsky, R., Matlin, N. & Jordaan, J.P. (1963). *Career development: Self-concept theory.* New York: College Entrance Examination Board.

Chapter 2

THEORETICAL FRAMEWORK AND REVIEW OF THE LITERATURE

The combining of art therapy with psychotherapy has received much attention in professional literature, often controversial because of "territorial" discipline issues. The match appears to be natural because of the combining of the cognitive domain with the affective, expressive domain. Psychotherapists have found that their clients vary greatly in their expressive styles, and allowing a modality that includes a full range of expression can more readily facilitate a variety of communication styles.

During the 1940s, Naumburg (1947) developed the use of art as a tool in psychotherapy. Her method was based on releasing the unconscious through spontaneous art expression. Her art therapy had its roots in the transference relationship between patient and therapist and the encouragement of free association. Naumburg stressed an extension of psychoanalysis and focused on intensive work with individual patients. Art therapy, as she defined it, was a primary therapeutic method.

A decade later, Kramer (1958) relied on psychoanalytic concepts and the later findings of Freudian ego psychology. She concentrated on the therapeutic values inherent in art. With this method, patients usually are seen in groups, and their art activities are an integral part of the therapeutic milieu. Kramer defined the goals of art therapy as those leading toward personality growth and rehabilitation. Later work by Kramer (1972) presented principles of interpretation of children's art and guidelines for the art therapist in which the therapeutic effect of art therapy is emphasized. More recently, Kramer and Wilson (1979) expressed the need for the art therapist to assist the client in the creative process, helping the client to draw using the client's own style and truths. In Kramer and Wilson's book, *Childhood and Art Therapy* (1979), the emphasis is on the idea of art as therapy, rather than on psychotherapy which uses art as a tool. Art therapy is conceived of primarily as a means of supporting the ego, fostering the development of a sense of identity, and promoting maturation in general. Its main function is seen in the power of art as a contributor to the development of psychic organization that is able to function under pressure without breakdown or the need to resort to stultifying defensive measures. So conceived, art therapy becomes both an essential component of the therapeutic milieu and a form of therapy that complements or supports psychotherapy but does not replace it.

Kramer's (Kramer & Wilson, 1979) extensive study of psychoanalysis helped her formulate many of her principles regarding the relationship between art and sublimation, aggression, and symbolism. *Sublimation* is a process wherein direct instinctive gratification is relinquished and a substitute activity is found that permits symbolic gratification of the same need in a socially productive way. An important feature of sublimation is the pleasure that the substitute activity affords. It can bind anxiety and aggression. However, the beneficial qualities of sublimation are limited. It is a defense mechanism based on renunciation of instinctive gratification. It is an advantageous compromise. If one accepts the theory of sublimation, it can be seen as an important factor in the artistic process.

Kwiatkowska is another therapist whose highly developed experience as an artist has been supplemented by clinical training. Her work in art evaluation and therapy with family groups provided a further development of the field in keeping with psychiatric trends of the 1960s and 1970s. Primary emphasis is placed on the development of immediate relationships among family members. Kwiatkowska was the first art therapist to introduce art therapy at a research center (National Institute of Mental Health) in 1958. Her patients participated in family art therapy as well as individual art therapy. The nursing staff, occupational therapists, and psychiatrists all participated in the research, which consisted of analytically oriented therapy serving as an adjunct to psychotherapy. Experiences with patients were presented and discussed at clinical conferences that included the entire staff. Her family art therapy approach has proven suitable for application in community mental health centers (1978).

Art therapy in the United States originated in connection with psychotherapy and the leading concepts derived from psychoanalytic theory. Art therapy has branched out from its original place in psychiatric hospitals to rehabilitation centers for the physically disabled, penal/correctional institutions, and special education schools.

In special education, progressive art educators adapted their techniques for the physically, mentally, and emotionally handicapped. Lowenfeld (1968) used the term "art education therapy" to define a therapy specific to the means of art education. Lowenfeld and associates' important work established baseline data on the art of normal children and has provided criteria for use when analyzing the art of emotionally or mentally disturbed clients.

Ulman (1975) formulated a synthesis of the psychoanalytic approaches expounded by Naumburg (1953) and Kramer (1972). Ulman defined the arts as a way of bringing order out of chaos, a means of discovering both the self and the world, and a means of establishing a relationship between the two. Like Kramer, Ulman also emphasized the healing quality of the creative process. But she also recognized that the completion of the artistic process may need to be sacrificed for more immediate goals; communication and insight may take priority over development of art expression.

Betensky (1973) promoted self-discovery through the arts and suggested that the creative process might be useful in the amelioration of psychological distress.

The philosophies and methods of modern art education both complement and parallel developments in modern psychology, psychotherapy, and psychoanalysis. Art education is now more flexible and adaptable to different needs, situations, and types of people. According to Kramer and Wilson (1979), the goal of all creative art teaching is to bring about the synthesis of emotional freedom and structured expression. The same principle remains the guiding idea also where creative activities serve more general goals of rehabilitation and therapy.

Wadeson (1980) approached psychotherapy as an educational process to help people with problems in living rather than as a treatment for a disease. Working primarily with adults, Wadeson saw the educational process as an effectually oriented facilitation of emotional growth rather than as a traditional cognitive model.

In 1981, McNiff related the integration of the arts and therapy as harking back to ancient methods of healing and stated that the emotional scope of art is unparalleled by other modes of expression. He saw the psychotherapeutic use of art as the integration of scientific knowledge about the psyche with the more imaginative and spiritual hemisphere of the mind, where the power to heal lies. McNiff presented the power of art in psychotherapy to be in art's ability to change, renew, and revalue the existing order.

The need for the integration of the spiritual dimension of the client with the more scientific method currently used by art therapists and other mental health professionals has been suggested by several researchers. Dufrene (1988), in her comparison of the traditional education of Native American healers with the education of American art therapists, recommended that therapists consider the spiritual dimension of the client during evaluation and treatment. She also recommended that researchers be more flexible in their adherence to the scientific method when research is conducted on topics that do not adhere to the scientific model, such as shamanic or traditional healing. McNiff (1981) also noted the similarities between shamanism and contemporary creative art therapies. He discussed the interconnections between shamanism and healing traditions and presented clinical examples of how symbolism and imaginal components of individuation occur in expressive art therapy.

The use of art, combined with psychotherapy, in the healing process is gaining widespread popularity and is being used more commonly. The range of art forms being utilized also is broadening. Jennings (1990) promoted dramatherapy, which emphasizes the art form of drama and theater as its central focus as a clinical and educational approach to gaining personal insight. Movement, art, and drama have been reported to bring about substantive gains in therapy when body image issues are being addressed, and masks and video have been used to facilitate interpersonal communication. Music also has been combined with other creative modalities in treatment.

Art therapy and psychotherapy are being used for an increasing range of experiences and with all age groups. Art has proven to be an important aid in the treatment of relationship problems. Blending psychotherapy with art therapy is an appropriate and effective way to evaluate and treat physically and sexually abused children. Young victims can express their feelings about abuse more easily through art. Art therapy also enables young victims to be more assertive and self-protective in both sexual and nonsexual situations (Hagood, 1991). Hagood believed that the parents, especially the mothers of the abused children, also may be able to function better by utilizing art to work through the crisis of abuse.

Therapists have found that post-session art making is useful for processing strong feelings, clarifying confused feelings, or giving form to unacknowledged feelings brought about by interaction with clients (Wadeson, 1989). Useful clinical information may be provided and empathy may increase with the therapist's use of post-session art.

Artistic creations sometimes reveal facets of personality not easily accessible through verbal psychotherapy. Important diagnostic indications may be discussed through free art expression before they can be identified by more conventional projective techniques. Symbolic content and the formal characteristics of the work constitute a source of information uniquely available through the visual arts.

Art therapists and psychotherapists have goals in common. One of those goals is to unite the powers of creativity and artistic freedom with the powers of a more rational frame of mind or intellect so that a more healthy, balanced person can emerge. In essence, this goal is to achieve a synthesis of a healthy unconscious and conscious mind through the innate creativity that is inherent at some level in all people. Art therapy brings unconscious material closer to the surface by providing an area of symbolic experience (Dufrene, 1988).

BIBLIOGRAPHY

McNiff, S. (1986). *Educating the creative arts therapist.* Springfield, IL: Charles C. Thomas.

Naumburg, M. (1973). *An introduction to art therapy: Studies of the "free" art expression of behavior problem children and adolescents as a means of diagnosis and therapy.* New York: Teachers College Press.

REFERENCES

Betensky, M. (1973). *Self-discovery through self-expression: Psychotherapy with children and adolescents.* Springfield, IL: Charles C. Thomas.

Dufrene, P.M. (1988). *A comparison of the traditional education of Native American healers with the education of the American art therapists.* Ann Arbor, MI: University Microfilms International.

Hagood, M. (1990). Group art therapy with mothers of sexually abused children. *The Arts in Psychotherapy, 18,* 17-27.

Jennings, S. (1990). *Dramatherapy with families, groups, and individuals: Waiting in the wings.* London: J. Kingsley.

Kramer, E. (1958). *Art therapy in a children's community: A study of art therapy in the treatment program of Wiltwyck School for Boys.* Springfield, IL: Charles C. Thomas.

Kramer, E. (1972). *Art as therapy with children.* New York: Schocken Books.

Kramer, E., & Wilson, L. (1979). *Childhood and art therapy: Notes on theory and application.* New York: Schocken Books.

Kwiatkowska, H.Y. (1978). *Family therapy and evaluation through art.* Springfield, IL: Charles C. Thomas.

Lowenfeld, V. (1968). *Viktor Lowenfeld speaks of art and creativity.* Washington, DC: National Art Education Association.

McNiff, S. (1981). *Arts and psychotherapy.* Springfield, IL: Charles C. Thomas.

Naumburg, M. (1947). *Studies of the "free" art expression of behavior problem children and adolescents as a means of diagnosis and therapy.* New York: Coolidge Foundation.

Naumburg, M. (1953). *Psychoneurotic art: Its function in psychotherapy.* New York: Grune and Stratton.

Ulman, E. (1975). *Art therapy in theory and practice.* New York: Schocken Books.

Wadeson, H. (1980). *Arts and psychotherapy.* Springfield, IL: Charles C. Thomas.

Wadeson, H. (1989). *Advances in art therapy.* New York: Wiley.

Chapter **3**

BLENDING ART THERAPY AND PSYCHOTHERAPY

Since art therapy is by nature interdisciplinary, encompassing art, psychology, and therapy, it is very common for alignments to occur between art therapists and more verbally oriented psychotherapists. Sometimes the alignment is compatible or complementary; other times it may be conflictual. Clients may receive treatment with both art therapists and psychotherapists in special education schools, hospitals, outpatient clinics, prisons, private practice offices, etc. As both art therapists and psychotherapists grow and develop, addressing new populations, both disciplines must work together to create new ways of using therapy for treatment and growth.

The blending of art therapy and psychotherapy, often called art psychotherapy or clinical art therapy, has its roots in the 1950s psychoanalytic theories and writings of Naumberg and Kramer that emphasized free association and sublimation (Landgarten, 1981; Wadeson, 1989). Art psychotherapy/clinical art therapy usually uses art therapy as the primary treatment and is considered effective for gaining awareness, reality testing, problem solving, revealing unconscious material, catharsis, solving conflicts, integration, and individuation (Landgarten, 1981).

People are attracted to art therapy because of its ability to merge interests in art and social service. Art therapy has the ability to be interdependent with the traditions of psychology and psychiatry, adapting to the language of the mental health professions (McNiff, 1986). The discipline of art therapy helps in the communication process with verbal psychotherapies, increases the possi-

13

bilities for interpersonal understanding, and is sometimes the only method of reaching individuals who are depressed, suffering from psychosis, withdrawn, etc. (McNiff, 1986).

Western psychotherapy is based on the premise that emotional conflicts can be resolved through rational analysis. Western oriented psychotherapists use dreams, free associations, and art to gather material for this rationalization. The creative process is used to heal the damaged psyche and facilitate the therapeutic relationship. Therapists who are too dependent on rational discourse place the art making process in a subordinate position to the intellectual discourse. According to McNiff, a more positive approach occurs through the following process:

> When talking in therapy proceeds poetically and imaginatively, within a story telling form, and when the relationship between therapist and client is an expression of the creative process, spoken language becomes artistic transformation. Therapy and art are concerned with transformative change, and the effective therapist is a person who is able to fully engage the creative resources of the environment. (1986, p. 9)

Rather than succumbing to an overreliance on Western rationalism to effect therapeutic change, clinical art therapy/art psychotherapy instead can rely on its foundation in the artistic process. However, this does not negate the necessity for art therapists who work closely with psychotherapists to be able to explain the art therapy process in a manner that is comprehensible within the prevailing mental health theoretical systems.

Art therapy can be interpreted from a Freudian, Jungian, or other theoretical orientation, but it is important to understand the client's own interpretation. Clinical art therapy helps clients record the therapeutic process through imagery and written commentary. Patients supplement art with thoughts, emotions, and free associations that are relevant to their productions. Experiences are shared visually and verbally. Techniques are presented that are pertinent to the needs of the individual and may be self-directed or may be topics recommended by the art therapist (Landgarten, 1981). Themes could include such things as wishes, dreams, fantasies, plans, family life, and one's environment. The art psychotherapist observes the client's creative process, the client's response to the art materials, and the elements/principles of the final art product to make appropriate diagnostic evaluations (Landgarten, 1981).

In some working situations, art psychotherapists work as primary therapists along with psychologists, clinical social workers, and other mental health personnel, providing individual and group therapy. In private practice, as in the case of the authors, the art therapist may work as an equal cotherapist in group therapy, as an adjunct therapist/consultant when verbal therapy is becoming "blocked," or as the primary therapist who at times uses the services of a psychologist for test administration. Successful art psychotherapy requires "interdependence with other mental health professionals in terms of theoretical understanding, communication, and operational methods" (McNiff, 1986, p. 133).

All therapists, regardless of orientation, must be able to respond empathetically with a variety of patient populations and situations. Therapy is a helping profession that requires sensitive, interpersonal skills. Therapy is an "art," not an exact science. Acknowledging therapy as an "art" reinforces acceptance of art into the therapeutic structure and facilitates the integration/blending of art and psychotherapy. Art's power to evaluate, intensify, increase, and clarify one's awareness is the key to the connection between clinical and artistic skills. A balanced integration of art and psychotherapy can be achieved by giving equal weight to both disciplines.

According to McNiff (1986), psychotherapists, artists, and art therapists all are concerned with understanding the self and others, environmental observations, relationships, and emotional changes. While artists are trained to express their emotions through sensory, creative processes, the clinician is lacking in this training, although it is a necessary skill in accessing emotions from clients. However, some of the most profound theories of psychology and psychiatry emanated from Jung and Freud, who were acutely sensitive to art's role in Western and non-Western cultures.

In order for the creative process to blend successfully with verbal psychotherapy and its goal of achieving self-actualization, art must be recognized as a vital component of life, across time and cultures. Art has the same goals as therapy: communication, catharsis, appreciation of life in all its dimensions, the expression of values and beliefs, and in non-Western forms of therapy, affirmation of spirituality.

The blending of art therapy and psychotherapy in primary treatment or adjunctive treatment is expanding to include populations with physiological disorders as well as psychological problems. This more holistic approach to treating physical as well as mental illness is particularly conducive to art psychotherapy/clinical art therapy and its integration of the emotional, spiritual, cognitive, and physical qualities of art. Art psychotherapy has the potential to be in the vanguard of effecting treatment changes in the health professions.

However, despite the differences and/or similarities in art therapy and psychotherapy, adherents to both modalities stress the necessity for the clinician to be adept in human understanding and interpersonal/intrapersonal relationships. This requires all types of therapists to be open to self-reflection and growth, constructive criticism, new forms of knowledge, and supervision as needed. Although not always recognized as a requirement for change by Western oriented therapists, acknowledgment and respect of higher powers is a major component of indigenous art and healing.

REFERENCES

Landgarten, H. (1981). *Clinical art therapy.* New York: Brunner/Mazel.

McNiff, S. (1986). *Educating the creative arts therapist.* Springfield, IL: Charles C. Thomas.

Wadeson, J. (Ed.). (1989). *Advances in art therapy.* New York: John Wiley & Sons.

Chapter 4

CASE STUDIES: CHILDREN AND ADOLESCENTS

The authors have worked individually and as cotherapists on a number of cases involving children and adolescents. In this chapter, utilizing the American Psychiatric Association (1994) *Diagnostic and Statistical Manual of Mental Disorders, Fourth Edition* (DSM-IV), the authors will outline several cases and how art therapy and psychotherapy were used to facilitate growth among clients. In order to protect the identity of clients, certain details have been changed.

CASE STUDY #1

Brief Historical Overview

This case involves two Caucasian siblings: a boy, Bill, and a girl, Mary, ages seven and eight respectively, abandoned by their welfare parents before ages one and two. Being wards of the state, the children were referred for counseling as they were being considered for adoption. At the writing of this book, the family discussed is continuing in treatment with both Coleman and Farris-Dufrene.

Mental Status Evaluation

These patients were oriented to the three spheres of person, time, and place; each had a broad affect. Both children were extremely intelligent and articulate.

The evaluation indicated that they had good recent and remote memory. School records revealed that both were at grade level, having good academic and behavioral assessments.

Empirical Observations

Assessed Psychological Impairment. Clinical assessments from projective instruments such as the *House, Tree, Person* (HTP) and other measures revealed that both children experienced trauma due to abandonment by their parents, particularly the mother; frequent foster home placements; fear of sibling separation; and possible physical/sexual assault. For example, prior to treatment provided by the authors, the results of the HTP indicated that the houses were drawn barren and lifeless, and figures had missing arms or legs, which often suggests clients' feelings of a lack of control, especially of their environment. Other measures, such as the *Kinetic Family Drawing Test* (KFD), often excluded parental figures, which may indicate the clients' response to abandonment and inability to accept the numerous foster parents as caretakers.

Disability Due to Impairment. Professional observations, including those of their pediatrician, guidance counselor, and school nurse, reported that the sister suffered from encopresis. Consequently, significant impairment was occurring in social, academic, and family relationships. The brother's records did not indicate any evidence of physiological impairment; therefore, his social interactions were age appropriate. Although normal sibling rivalry was prevalent, it was exacerbated by the sister's day and night urine emissions.

Diagnosis (Per the DSM-IV)

Mary/Sister

Axis I—Posttraumatic Stress Disorder, 309.81
    Adjustment Disorder with Depressed Mood, 309.00
Axis II—799.99, Diagnosis Deferred
Axis III—Encopresis (No physiological basis)
Axis IV—Psychosocial and Environmental Problems: Separation Anxiety, Depression, Abandonment
    Severity: Moderate to Severe
Axis V—Current GAF: 60 (moderate symptoms)
    Highest GAF Past Year: 50 (serious symptoms)
    Previous GAF Prior to Counseling: 40 (impairment in communication, family, and school relations)

Bill/Brother

Axis I—Posttraumatic Stress Disorder, 309.81
   Adjustment Disorder with Depressed Mood, 309.00
Axis II—799.99, Diagnosis Deferred
Axis III—None
Axis IV—Psychosocial and Environmental Problems: Separation Anxiety, Depression, Abandonment
   Severity: Moderate
Axis V—Current GAF: 80 (transient and expectable reactions to stressors)
   Highest GAF Past Year: 60 (moderate symptoms)
   Previous GAF Prior to Counseling: 50 (serious symptoms, impairment in impulse control)

Nellie/Adoptive Mother

Axis I—Depressive Disorder, Nos, 311.00
   Adjustment Disorder with Depressed Mood, 309.00
Axis II—799.90, Diagnosis Deferred
Axis III—Migraine Headaches
Axis IV—Psychosocial and Environmental Problems: Parenting, Life Transition, Depression
   Severity: Moderate to Severe
Axis V—Current GAF: 65 (mild symptoms)
   Highest GAF Past Year: 55 (moderate difficulty in social, occupational functioning)
   Previous GAF Prior to Counseling: 55 (moderate difficulty in social, occupational functioning)

Arthur/Adoptive Father

Axis I—Adjustment Disorder with Anxiety, 309.24
Axis II—799.90, Diagnosis Deferred
Axis III—Obesity
Axis IV—Psychosocial and Environmental Problems: Parenting, Coping with Wife's Depression
   Severity: Moderate
Axis V—Current GAF: 85 (minimal symptoms and expectable reactions to psychosocial stressors)
   Highest GAF Past Year: 90 (minimal symptoms)
   Previous GAF Prior to Counseling: 85 (minimal symptoms)

Systems Impact

Because some impairment was present in the clients' functioning, this had a deleterious effect on their social adjustment to family and occasionally school situations. Both sister and brother expressed doubts as to the permanency of their pending adoption; doubts were manifested in their inappropriate behavior.

Treatment Plan

Treatment Modalities. Individual and family art and psychotherapy were provided on a biweekly basis for three years. The authors will summarize the treatment process through termination.

Introduction. While the traditional "talk therapy" provided sufficient information during the initial phases of treatment, it became apparent that additional techniques or approaches would be necessary in order to uncover the suspected physical/sexual abuse from the previous foster placements. The psychotherapist met with the parents to discuss the possibility of introducing an art therapy consultant, and the parents were quite receptive because they also had felt frustrated with respect to progress in therapy. It was decided that Coleman (psychotherapist) and Farris-Dufrene (art therapist) would function as cotherapists.

Initial Session. The cotherapists met with Bill and Mary, and discussed how subsequent sessions would be conducted. The clients were quite receptive to the addition of a new person and a new modality. Most of the first session was spent establishing rapport and setting the agenda for techniques and activities to be introduced. Both children were lively and animated and had no difficulty adapting to the new therapeutic environment.

During the initial art therapy sessions, the clients were allowed to choose their own theme for drawing. The purpose of this was to empower the children in order for them to identify the most important issues and themes in their lives. The drawing instruments chosen were colored felt-tip pens and white paper of assorted sizes. Mary tended to work more carelessly, constantly chattering while drawing, and interrupting her brother. Bill was quiet, engaged in his work, and had a longer attention span. Bill resented Mary's intrusions into his space while involvement in creative endeavors.

Mary. Although 8 years old, Mary tended to draw immature stick figures usually seen in much younger children. Knowing that she had an average IQ and exhibited above average intelligence, the art therapist encouraged her to draw fuller figures. When prompted, Mary could draw a human figure that was more age appropriate. One of her first drawings was of her and her adopted mother (Figure 1). A line drawn down the middle of the page separated her and her mother, with herself drawn much larger and more colorful than her mother. Subsequent therapy sessions revealed a rivalry between mother and daughter, which also had been addressed in previous sessions with the parents.

In a drawing of her house, a large dollar sign was illustrated on the second story of the home, with an arrow pointing to the second floor (Figure 2). The caption by the arrow stated "This is My House." In dialogues with the cotherapist while she drew the house, she compared her previous foster homes in depressed communities with her new house in a wealthy suburb. The title of Mary's picture was "Sit in the Back Yard." Five immature stick figures were drawn, as well as a car. The picture was drawn hastily, with little coloring or shading.

Other family pictures dealt with problems in previous foster homes. When discussing family issues, Mary vacillated between her adopted family and her previous foster homes. Both Coleman and Farris-Dufrene were concerned about possible abuse in the foster homes, which could have caused some of the present problems, such as encopresis. Like her first picture of herself and her mother, in another picture Mary drew a line down the middle of the page, separating her "bad" foster sister from the "good" foster sister. On the right side of the paper, the word "bad" was enclosed in a tulip shape, and the left side of the page had the word "good" enclosed in the same tulip shape. Her right side symbolized a former foster sister named Dianna. Dianna was portrayed with a large blue head, tears streaming down her face, an extremely long neck and shoulders, with a mouth turned upside down exposing two front teeth. The left represented the "good" foster sister named Beth. Mary also described herself as the figure. Beth/Mary was drawn as a cheerleader in brightly colored clothing. Mary mentioned that she would like Beth to visit her in her new adopted home. Mary also expressed fears of ever seeing the other foster sister, who Mary alluded to abusing her.

Interestingly, Mary compartmentalized her pictures, with herself on the left side and the others, often negative figures, on the right. In her pictures, seldom is contact shown between people. This may suggest how her transient lifestyle has been compartmentalized with respect to relationships with her biological parents, foster parents and siblings, adopted parents, and biological brother.

One of the primary issues in Mary's treatment was her encopresis and its repercussions in her social and family interactions. Mary, along with her par-

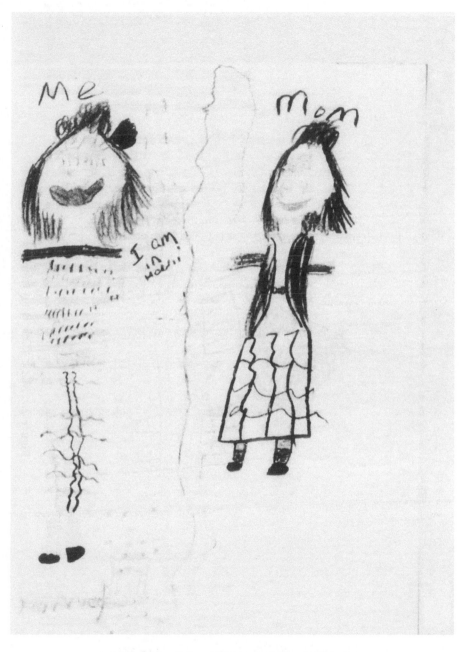

Figure 1.   Mary: "Me and Mom" (18" × 24").

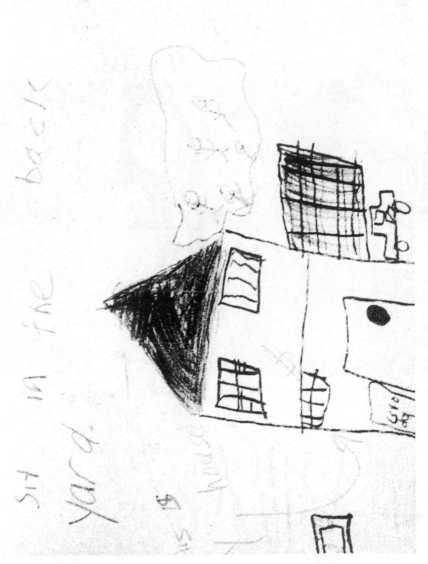

Figure 2. Mary: "This is my house" (18" × 24").

ents, had spent numerous sessions discussing the mother's frustration and Mary's embarrassment concerning this issue. The art therapist suggested that Mary explore this problem through art. Mary drew a series of pictures dealing with morning routines centered around using the bathroom. The pictures were done in a storyboard/cartoon format with captions. One series concerned household bathroom issues. One caption said, "First I get up and go to the bathroom, and if someone is in the bathroom, I knock on the door." The adjacent caption stated, "Then I get dressed," and showed her getting dressed. Mary's other picture dealt with school bathroom issues. In a drawing compartmentalized in three major sections, the top section illustrated a girls bathroom and a boys bathroom, with toilet stools in each bathroom. In the middle of the paper, the bathroom scene is titled, "Go to the bathroom." At the bottom of the page, is the last part of the bathroom series. These drawings were all sparse and sketchy, with minimal details. Mary had indicated verbally that she "soiled her underwear" on a daily basis while at school. To the dismay of her parents, especially her mother, Mary became oppositional with her parents and teachers, blaming her difficulties on not having enough time to get to the bathroom or the bathroom being in use by others. The issue of encopresis and soiling underwear frequently had become a source of consternation for the entire family.

Bill. Bill's artwork revealed a rich imagination, complex details, and figures that were fully developed. He preferred to work quietly, in his own space. One of his first pictures was titled, "My Mom and Dad are King and Queen of the World" (Figure 3). His parents were drawn with crowns on their heads and long robes. In the opinion of the art therapist, this image reflects Bill's view of his parents as rulers with power who will provide for the family, have control over their lives, and rescue him and his sister from the harm of their previous foster homes. Another picture is titled, "Mary and Bill are the Princess and Prince" (Figure 4). Bill and Mary are drawn with crowns on their heads, smiling faces, and outstretched arms. However, on the back of the picture Bill wrote, "Will you shut your mouth for the rest of day, Mary." The front of the page suggests compatibility and a congenial relationship, while the back of the page reveals some conflict. Coleman, in previous therapy sessions, had identified the issue of Mary's domination of Bill and his assertive responses.

When requested to draw a *House, Tree, Person,* Bill drew a tall, phallic shaped tree, with red apples, and green grass bordering the bottom of the page (Figure 5). The multicolored house (green, grey, blue, purple) is floating in space. Two boys are portrayed playing together; one is "King Bill" and the other is his friend, also named Bill. A little brown house is in the corner, identified as the friend's house. The phallic shaped tree possibly could indicate exposure and/or interest in sexual matters, or a normal male child's concern

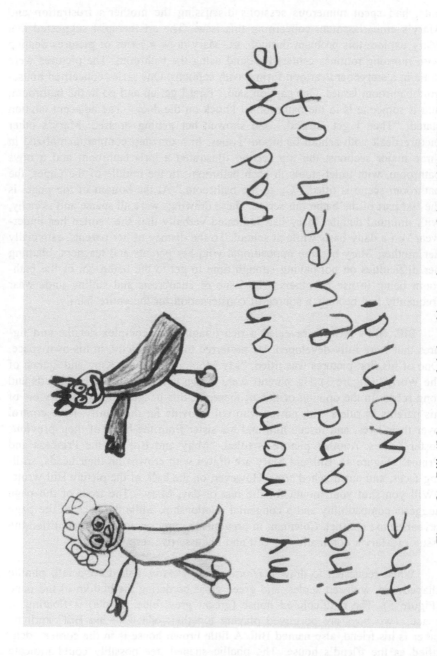

Figure 3. Bill: "My mom and dad are king and queen of the world" (18" × 24").

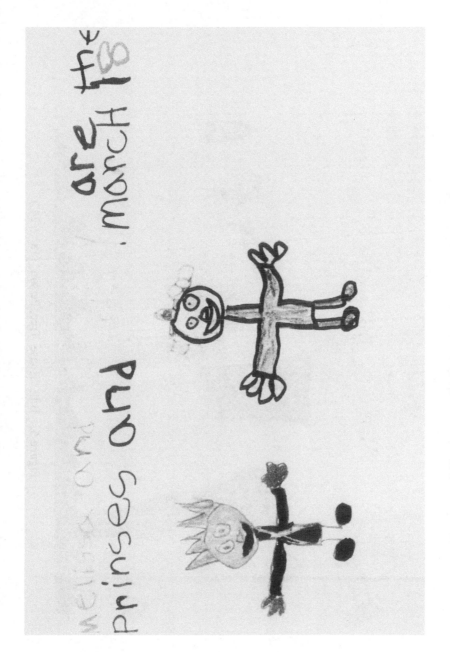

Figure 4. Bill: "Mary and Bill are the princess and prince" (18" × 24").

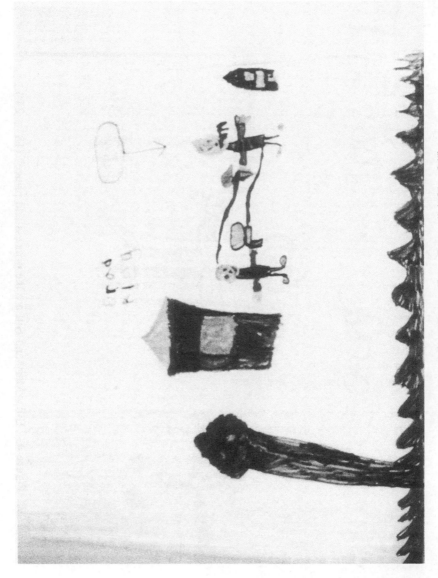

Figure 5. Bill: "House, Tree, Person" (18" × 24").

about his penis. The floating house may suggest the frequent foster placements, indicating no stability or grounding in the home. On the positive side, the house has windows and a door, is brightly colored and large, and overshadows the smaller house of his friend. It appears that Bill takes pride in his home, even though he may have insecurities about its permanency.

Some of Bill's other pictures included family and friends, brightly colored, with smiling faces and outstretched arms, various types of animals, and a series of dragons. One dragon figure, hugely drawn, had a blue and green tail spewing fire at a boy in the corner of the page (Figure 6). Other fantasy figures included a large, brown figure divided into quadrants, with green and blue arms and limbs and an open mouth with sharp, pointed, exposed teeth. He described these as cartoon characters, one of which is a Ninja Turtle (Figure 7). No evidence of pathology was seen in these dragon and other fantasy drawings. Although some may interpret the teeth and fire as violent imagery, it must be remembered that these are typical cartoon caricatures reflective of contemporary society. To detect whether these "violent" scenes are just television imagery or indications of personal violent experiences is often difficult. However, Bill, unlike Mary, was reluctant to discuss any possible previous abuse.

Parents. The adoptive parents had been married for 20 years and were unable to conceive despite genetic counseling. At the time of Nellie and Arthur's consideration of adoption, the agency could not identify a Caucasian infant. Their options were a minority infant, a special needs infant or child, or older children. After much consternation and deliberation, the couple decided to adopt an older child. However, most older children had siblings also in need of adoption. It was during this time that Nellie and Arthur became foster parents for two prospective adoptees, Bill and Mary.

Because the couple had been childless for so many years, tremendous adjustments to their lifestyle were needed. The transition to parenthood was exacerbated by Nellie's chronic depression. During this difficult time of adjustment, the children's biological mother finally consented to adoption. It was at the stage of adoption finalization that the couple sought family counseling.

The psychotherapist developed a treatment plan that included individual and group counseling for the children, and family/couples counseling for the parents. The parents' adjustment to the children was causing marital problems, primarily because little or no time was available for the parents to be together after having spent over 20 years alone with each other. Arthur had more appropriate coping mechanisms and seemed to enjoy spending time with the children; however, Nellie became jealous of Arthur's attention being diverted from

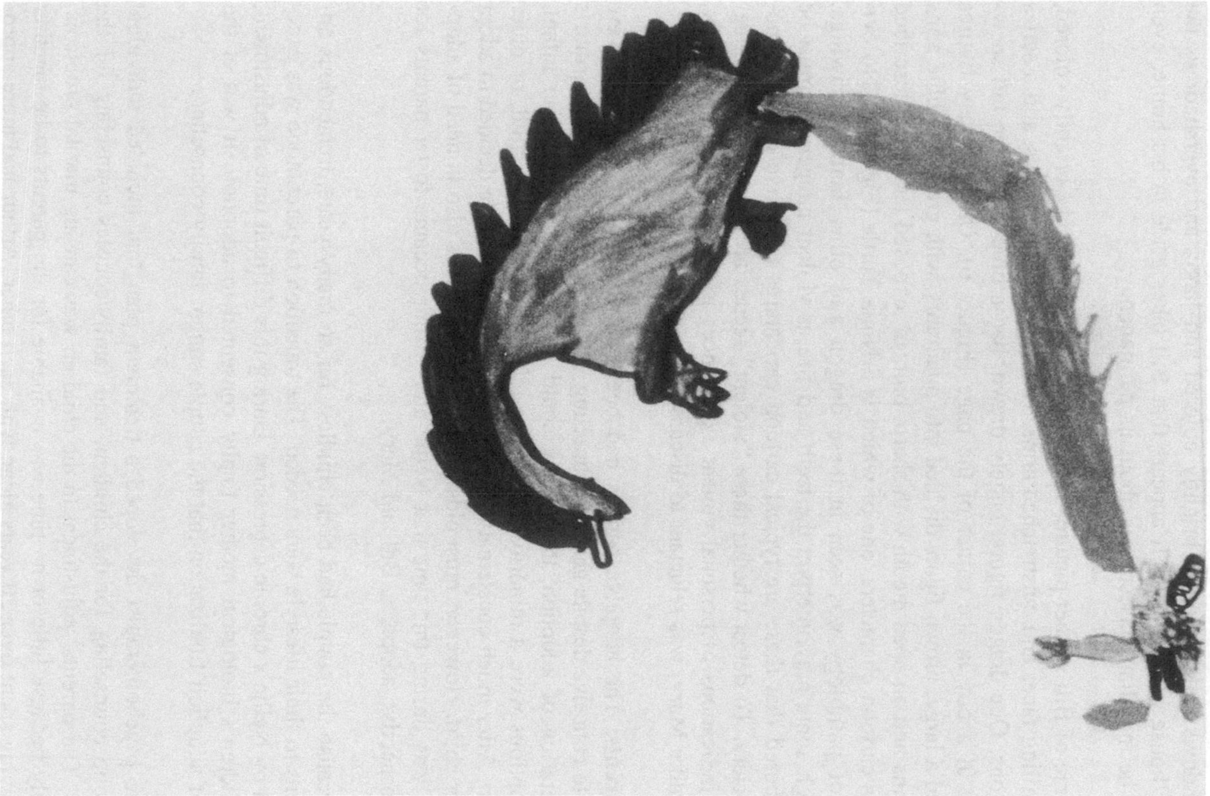

Figure 6. Bill: "Dragon" (18" × 24").

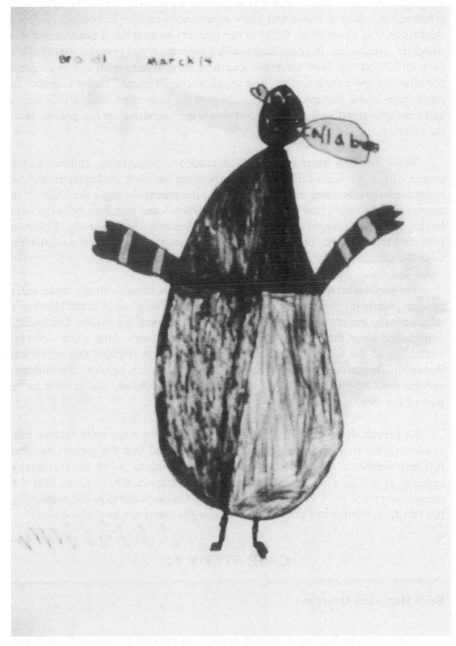

Figure 7. Bill: "Ninja Turtle" (18" × 24").

her to the children. Arthur and Bill were able to develop a positive father-son relationship, where as Nellie and Mary experienced conflict in bonding. Nellie's depression was a significant factor in her inability to establish a positive mother-daughter relationship. In consultation with Coleman, it was revealed that Nellie's own childhood had been traumatic due to sibling rivalry with her two sisters for attention from their mother. The psychotherapist invited Nellie's mother to participate in the therapeutic process, hoping to gain more insight into issues and concerns about Nellie's childhood that were impacting on her present family situation.

Nellie, and to a lesser extent Arthur, tended to perceive the children as the source of her problems rather than acknowledge her own inadequacies and be receptive to professional intervention. Thus, the parents brought the children to counseling indicating that they were the "problem" and that their behavior was having an adverse impact on the marital relationship. Subsequently, Coleman provided treatment for both children for two years with frequent consultation with the parents.

The psychotherapist apparently had reached an impasse in the therapeutic process. While the therapist felt that progress was being made in the children's adjustment to the adoption and the new family situation, the parents continually complained about the children's behavior and other issues. After a more careful evaluation of the family dynamics, the psychotherapist decided that additional therapeutic modalities might facilitate a better interaction between the children and parents. At this point, an art therapist, Farris-Dufrene, was invited to be part of the treatment team.

As previously mentioned, the parents and children were quite receptive to expanding the treatment team. However, it appeared that the parents resisted full involvement in the art therapy process, preferring to utilize the art therapy sessions as private time for themselves. Both therapists felt, at times, that the parents were not truly committed to sharing the responsibility for improving the family dynamics and only wanted to use the therapists as "baby-sitters."

CASE STUDY #2

Brief Historical Overview

Farris-Dufrene has had extensive experience providing services for children who have been sexually abused. In her work as an art therapist at a psychiatric hospital, most of the clients referred to her were sexually abused children. These children usually came from families with a history of physical and sexual abuse. This case study will explore the interrelationships and dynamics of three sisters who were sexually abused by their stepfather and grandfather, and physically abused by their biological father. Through art therapy, the sisters were able to articulate visually their feelings about their abusive environment.

Mental Status Evaluation

During the initial therapy sessions, the youngest child, Anne, age 7, rocked herself and crouched in a fetal position on the floor. She sucked her thumb and was noncommunicative. Andrea, her 8-year-old sister, presented sexually acting out behavior and was sexually provocative toward male staff. Nancy, the eldest sister, age 9, was the most verbal and tended to intellectualize her experiences.

Empirical Observations

Assessed Psychological Impairment. Clinical assessment and evaluation revealed that the youngest and older sisters' experience of being sexually abused meet the criteria for Posttraumatic Stress Disorder as delineated in the DSM-IV. Although the younger child had evidence of physical abuse, it was inconclusive as to whether or not she also had been abused sexually; however, she still exhibited severe psychological disorders.

Disability Due to Impairment. The two younger children had academic difficulties in school, such as hyperactivity, disruptive behavior, and low grades. But the oldest child performed well academically until the abuse was reported, at which time her grades also became lower. The two youngest children also were involved in stealing from teachers and neighbors.

Diagnosis (Per the DSM-IV)

Anne

Axis I—Posttraumatic Stress Disorder, 309.81
    Adjustment Disorder with Depressed Mood, 309.00
Axis II—799.90, Diagnosis Deferred
Axis III—None
Axis IV—Psychosocial and Environmental Problems: Social and Academic Impairment
    Severity: Severe

Axis V—Current GAF: 60 (difficulty in social and academic functioning)
Highest GAF Past Year: 60
Previous GAF Prior to Incident: 60

Andrea

Axis I—Posttraumatic Stress Disorder, 309.81
Adjustment Disorder with Depressed Mood, 309.00
Axis II—799.99, Diagnosis Deferred
Axis III—Evidence of Bruised Genitalia, Taking Ritalin
Axis IV—Psychosocial and Environmental Problems: Hyperactivity, Social and Academic Impairment
Axis V—Current GAF: 60 (difficulty in social and academic functioning)
Highest GAF Past Year: 60
Previous GAF Prior to Incident: 60

Nancy

Axis I—Posttraumatic Stress Disorder, 309.81
Adjustment Disorder with Depressed Mood, 309.00
Axis II—799.99, Diagnosis Deferred
Axis III—None
Axis IV—Psychosocial and Environmental Problems: Social and Academic Impairment
Axis V—Current GAF: 60 (difficulty in social and academic functioning)
Highest GAF Past Year: 60
Previous GAF Prior to Incident: 60

Systems Impact

The three sisters all are experiencing adjustment problems at school, in the community, and at home. This interferes with their academic performance, ability to interact appropriately with neighbors, and overall psychosocial development.

Review of the Literature

Sexual abuse is a widespread phenomenon inflicted on children by adults in authoritative positions, usually children's own guardians (Manning, 1987). Since the 1960s, the public has been made more aware of this national tragedy, and legislation has been enacted to protect child sexual abuse victims. Psychiatric exploration of child abuse, psychological studies of abusive parents, and art therapy case studies of child abuse originated in the early 1960s (Manning, 1987).

Although child physical and/or sexual abuse is known to be a widespread tragedy, reliable statistics really do not exist. Consequently, the research is inconclusive. For example, some researchers estimate 100,000–500,000 annual cases, others indicate 20 million Americans, and others even report figures of 60,000–4,000,000 (Sidun, 1987). One of the reasons for the various numerical discrepancies is fear and shame of disclosure (Sidun, 1987).

According to art therapists and other mental health and educational specialists, art therapy is the most appropriate and least stressful technique for diagnosis and treatment of child abuse victims (Powell, 1990). Children are more comfortable drawing pictures related to traumatic events than verbalizing about such experiences.

Group art therapy is often the most effective method because interaction with other abused children lessens feelings of isolation and helps child victims share their experiences. Powell and other art therapists (Hagood, 1991; Manning, 1987; Serrano, 1989; Sidun, 1987) have said that not being believed can be more traumatic than the actual abuse. By sharing sexual abuse experiences in a group, children receive support and confirmation.

Of prime importance is clarification of the sexual offense as an abuse of power by the adult perpetrator. Child sexual abuse victims need clarification of each person's role in the sexual offense and treatment, including their own roles as victims, roles of their guardians and/or perpetrator, roles of the police and/or court investigators, and the role of the therapist.

Hagood (1991) and Powell (1990) mentioned the necessity for parents of abused children (particularly the mothers) to have therapy. Improvement of the mother's emotional well- being may permit the entire family to function better. The whole family is in crisis when incest and/or abuse is reported. Family therapy can improve the parenting skills of dysfunctional families.

According to Hagood, art therapy uncovers unconscious feelings and problems about the abuse and family dynamics that may not be evident in a verbal exchange. A common task is for clients to portray graphically their relationships with their mothers and other family members (including the abuser). Other art therapy techniques include self-portraits to measure the client's self-image, drawing pictures of positive and negative feelings about the abuser, puppetry with anatomically correct dolls to clarify boundary issues related to appropriate and inappropriate touching, and working with clay to release angry feelings through pounding and squeezing (Powell, 1990).

Sexual abuse occurrences in children are often difficult to detect and/or diagnose through traditional verbal assessments such as intake interviews. Art therapists and psychologists often use the *D-A-P* (*Draw A Person*) instrument to detect child sexual abuse. The *D-A-P (Draw A Person)* test is nonintrusive because it makes minimal verbal demands on the child. Because offenders frequently threaten physical harm to the child if he or she reports the abuse, sexually abused children and adolescents view verbal psychotherapy as intimidating.

Researchers report conflicting results in identifying graphic indicators of sexual abuse. Some hypothesize that sexually abused children and adolescents draw more oversized and oversexualized people than do nonabused children and adolescents. Oversexualized features could be excessive hair, overly emphasized open mouth, the presence of breasts, drawing the trouser fly, shading genital areas, and hands covering the genital area (Sidun, 1987). It also is hypothesized that abused children draw more triangular shaped wedges, phallic shapes, and circles. Other features are omitted eye pupils and omitted hands and fingers. Researchers speculate that the omission of hands and fingers is related to feelings of guilt, vulnerability, helplessness, and perceptions of bodily damage.

However, these graphic indicators are not prevalent in all cases and may be present in the drawings of nonabused children and adolescents. Sidun (1987) cautioned that adolescent sexual interest is normal, and sexually graphic features are not always proof of abuse. Studies of the drawings of abused and nonabused adolescents may be helpful to clinicians in alerting them to the possibility of sexual abuse. However, it is also necessary to explore the adolescent's family and sexual history.

Art produces a concrete visual image of the abuse problem. A commonality among victims is a distorted body image, an image of the body as ugly or as separated from the head through color or space. Eventually, abuse victims become more aware of their fractured parts, the absence of legs or arms, and the sense of isolation evident in their art. This awareness is a step toward recovery (Serrano, 1989).

Art therapy helps victims express and resolve feelings regarding the abuse, enabling them to be more assertive and self-protective in sexual situations. Treatment is a long process, often lasting two years or more. It is important that children realize that at some future point in their lives they may need further treatment related to the abuse.

Treatment Plan

Initially, Anne, Andrea, and Nancy were referred for group therapy for sexually abused children as well as family therapy. The two youngest children did not respond to verbal therapy and were unwilling to disclose. Family therapy was unsuccessful due to the mother's noncompliance with the treatment process.

Treatment Modalities—Introduction. Because of the younger children's inability to respond to verbal therapy, they were invited to join an art therapy group for sexually abused children. All three sisters were involved in this therapeutic process, along with three sexually abused boys. Eventually, the boys were discharged from the hospital, and the girls continued in treatment. The girls also were seen individually by the art therapist.

Anne. Anne is a 7-year-old white female with brown hair and brown eyes. This was her first psychiatric hospitalization. Anne is described by her mother and school officials as hyperactive, disruptive, and inattentive. She had been caught stealing from teachers. Born premature, Anne had a pinched aorta at birth, which required heart surgery when Anne was 6 months old. There is no evidence of sexual abuse by the stepfather. But Anne had reported that her father "beat me and my sisters and made red marks on my arms and legs."

Andrea. Andrea is a white female with red hair and brown eyes. Andrea was diagnosed with Attention Deficit Disorder in 1990 by a community health clinic. The client took Ritalin for six months until her mother went off Medicaid and could not afford the medication. Her mother reported that Andrea's behavior problems began at age 4 with stealing from the neighbors. Andrea's mother also reported that her daughter sat on the couch, rocking herself, and humming. The client was discovered lying naked on top of her 6-year-old sister. The mother reported that Andrea masturbated at night. She also was discovered nude in the back seat of a car kissing a boy her age. Her school grades are poor, and teachers reported that she was disruptive, defiant, and destructive to property. Through a gynecological examination, there was evidence of sexual abuse and bruised genitalia. Andrea implicated her stepfather in the abuse. Andrea also had been abused physically by the biological father, resulting in welts on her buttocks from beatings.

Nancy. Nancy is a 9-year-old white female with brown hair and brown eyes. Nancy lies and steals at home and in the neighborhood. However, she had good behavior in school. But in the last year, her grades have dropped from A's and B's to D's and F's. The mother worried about Nancy's promiscuous behavior. The mother reported that Nancy puts on "see-through" nightgowns or miniskirts and climbs all over her grandfather's lap. The mother reported that the grandfather abused Nancy when she was a child. Regarding any sexual abuse between the client and her stepfather, the client had given conflicting messages.

The family history involves divorce, remarriage, alcohol problems, and periods of unemployment and welfare dependency. Because of employment instability with the husband, the mother and five children have moved several times. Although the youngest daughter and oldest daughter also have been sexual abuse victims, they were not admitted for psychiatric hospitalization. At various times, the children have lived in foster homes while their mother was treated for depression and child neglect.

Art Therapy Sessions. The three sisters attended their first art therapy group for sexual abuse. The group originally included three boys who had been sexually molested by their fathers/stepfathers, but due to an early discharge for the three boys and extended hospitalization for the sisters, the group eventually consisted of only the three siblings. The activity for the first session included drawing or painting a self-portrait, followed by a family portrait. Anne cried about the way her pictures looked, tore them, and threw them away. Nancy was reluctant to draw or paint but eventually participated. Andrea was also displeased with her artwork and threw her drawings away. All three girls experienced confusion in deciding who to include in a family portrait. Discussions revolved around whether or not to draw the stepfather, biological father, or stepmother.

The following week we expanded the theme of self-portraiture to include the entire body drawn life-size. After the girls had traced each other's bodies on large paper, they were encouraged to draw and color their facial features, clothes, and body parts. There was a group discussion about which part of the human body was private and should only be touched by a doctor versus body parts that could be touched by friends or relatives. We discussed "good touch," such as a hug or kiss on the cheek versus "bad touch," such as fondling someone's genital area.

Anne, the youngest sister, originally drew herself with short hair and pants (Figure 8). It was hard to determine if the figure was male or female. She then

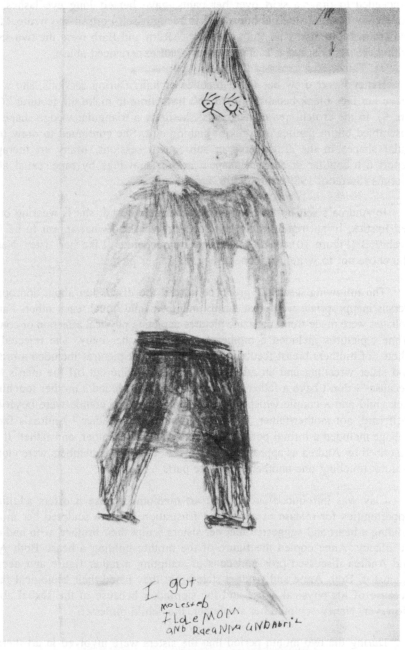

I got
molested
I late MOM
aNd RaeaNiva aNDAbriL

Figure 8.   Anne: "Self-portrait" (5' height).

proceeded to draw a skirt over her pants, gave herself long eye lashes, and added long hair. At the bottom of her full-length self-portrait she wrote, "I got molested. I tole mom and Ruth and Barb." Ruth and Barb were the two sisters who were not hospitalized, although they had experienced abuse.

Nancy never drew her facial features or hair. During sessions, she would leave her face blank because she "didn't have time to make the features" (Figure 9). In the crotch area of her pants, she drew a triangular wedge shape that resembled bikini panties or a bikini bathing suit. She continued to draw triangular shapes in the crotch area in subsequent sessions. Many art therapists report a triangular or vaginal shaped area in drawings by rape/sexual abuse victims (Serrano, 1989; Sidun, 1987).

In Andrea's self-portrait, her hair is long and blond; she is wearing bright red lipstick, bright red and purple clothes, gloves, and what appear to be false eyelashes (Figure 10). Her figure is most precocious. Like her sister, Nancy, she chose not to write a statement or title for her picture.

The following week the group continued the discussion about appropriate versus inappropriate ways that family members may touch each other. Family collages were made from magazine pictures depicting physical affection or contact. Anne's pictures included a mother bottle-feeding her baby. She rejected the photos of mothers breast-feeding their babies. Other pictures included a brother and sister wrestling and an adult couple hugging. She cut off the man's head because "I don't have a father." Nancy's pictures included a mother touching a sick child and a couple whispering. She stated that the couple were boyfriend/girlfriend, not mother/father, because "I don't have a father." Andrea's family collage included a formal portrait of a brother, sister, mother, and father. It was described by Andrea as appropriate because all the family members were clothed and not touching one another's "private parts."

Clay was introduced as the next art medium because it offers additional opportunities for release of anger and frustration. Andrea sculpted her mother holding a heart and suggested that her sisters sculpt their brother, who had died in infancy. Anne copied the figure of the mother holding a heart. Both Anne and Andrea discussed pros and cons of sculpting a father figure and decided against it. Both Anne and Andrea stated that they hated their biological father because of his physical abuse and the stepfather because of the sexual abuse. However, Nancy sculpted her stepfather, the "child molester."

During the two-month period that the sisters were involved in art therapy, the most memorable and illuminating sessions were those involving a series of

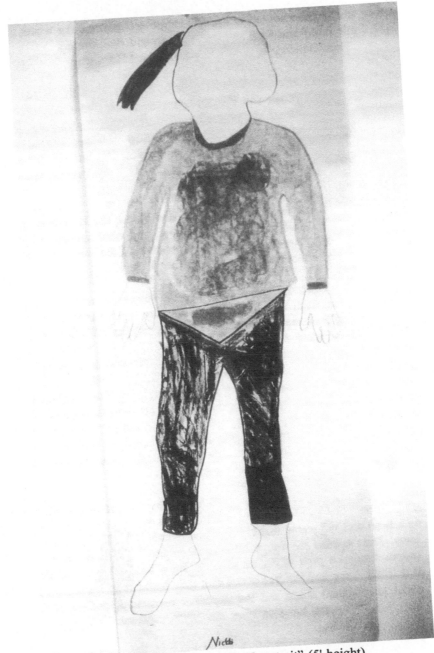

Figure 9.   Nancy: "Self-portrait" (5' height).

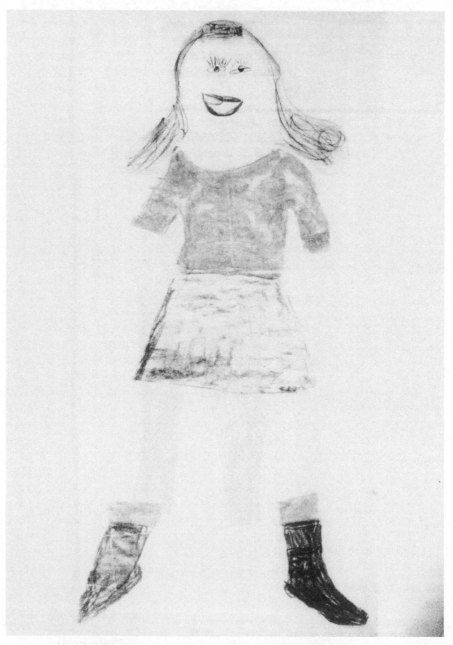

Figure 10. Andrea: "Self-portrait" (5' height).

murals depicting their stepfather's sexual abuse trial and a series on how to prevent sexual abuse. These murals served educational as well as therapeutic purposes. They subsequently were used to inform young children of ways to prevent possible abuse and of the necessity to disclose abuse if it should occur. Children exposed to these murals are thus better prepared to cope with social realities.

Some of the titles the girls chose were "I Don't Like to be Molested," "I Don't Want to be Molested Again," and "Being Molested is Nasty" (see Figure 11). The drawings depicted adult figures/strangers offering candy to children, children saying "no" to sexual advance, and strangers knocking on house doors while children are home alone.

While exploring the theme of sexual abuse prevention, the oldest sister was the most agitated, covering her ears with her hands while her sisters graphically described the sexual incidents. Nancy felt it was too "nasty" to talk about. In her picture, Nancy illustrated herself with her tongue sticking out and the recurring triangular shape in the crotch area. The caption near the girl's mouth says, "How would you like to be molested?" Another girl answers "No!"

To help the sisters prepare for the possibility of having to attend a trial or court hearing and the possibility that their stepfather might be incarcerated, Farris-Dufrene initiated mural themes on a sexual abuse trial. During the mural sessions, the two younger sisters expressed their anger towards the stepfather by fantasizing that he would be jailed for a long time and suffer beatings while incarcerated. They wanted their stepfather to be punished for causing their hospitalization. Both younger sisters felt that by disclosing their sexual abuse they had been punished with hospitalization. However, Nancy, the older sister, felt that the stepfather should have therapy instead of a prison sentence.

One mural scene is titled "20 to 60 Years" (Figure 12a). The stepfather, dressed in a striped prison uniform and a down-turned mouth, is standing next to the judge's bench. The female judge asks the young girl "Did he?" and she replies "Yes!" Another scene is titled "He's Going to be in Jail for 20 to 100 Years" (Figure 12b). The stepfather, dressed in a striped prison shirt, asks for help. The young girl replies, "I can't and I won't help you." All five sisters are standing next to the mother as she tells the judge, "That's what they told me."

Working on this mural series elicited information that was partly responsible for the sisters' transfer to a foster home. The sisters informed Farris-Dufrene that their mother had told them to tell the court that they did not remember the

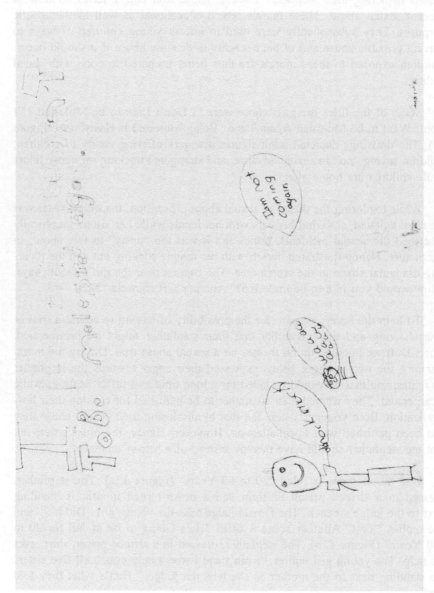

Figure 11. Andrea: "I don't want to be molested again" (18" × 24").

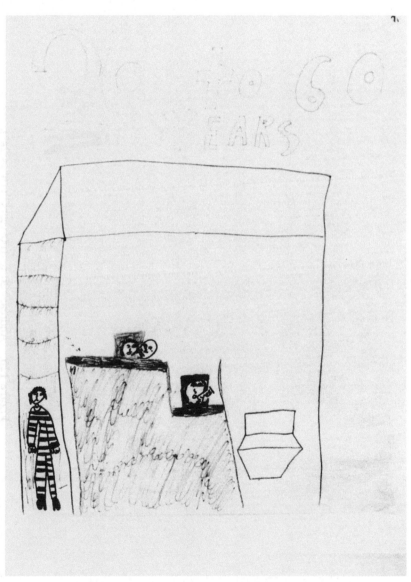

Figure 12a.   Andrea: "20 to 60 years" (18" × 24").

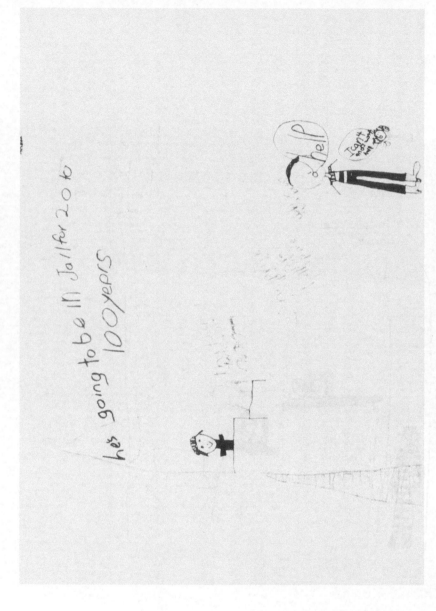

Figure 12b. Andrea: "20 to 100 years" (18" × 24").

45

molestation and had been lying. It was revealed that the mother defied the Child Protective Services by allowing the stepfather to remain in the house when the daughters had weekend visitations. The mural series also prompted conversations about molestation by the grandfather, and their mother's advice not to disclose it to prevent the grandfather from being arrested. Disclosure about the mother's desire not to have her husband incarcerated and allowing him to have contact with her children was corroborated in verbal psychotherapy sessions, resulting in neglect charges and a foster placement recommendation.

The concluding art therapy sessions dealt with termination of therapy, preparation for transfer to a foster home, and more educational and preventive measures. The sisters were introduced to the child's book, *My Body Is Private* (Girard, 1984), which describes a young girl's positive and negative reaction to certain types of touching by parents, siblings, a doctor, and an uncle. The girls illustrated scenes from that book and other children's books that covered themes such as divorce and physical abuse (Figure 13). Activities such as listening to therapeutic theme stories and illustrating them are appropriate for teachers, parents, and the lay public in general as preventive abuse measures.

Summary

This case highlights the difficulties of working with child abuse victims when the perpetrators are family members and there is a lack of cooperation from the nonabusive parent. It also illustrates the complexities of interfacing with the judicial, school, and social service systems. Often in cases such as these, the mission, goals, and objectives of the aforementioned agencies and families may be in direct conflict with the goals of therapeutic intervention. In order to adapt to these potential obstacles, therapists must be flexible, while concurrently maintaining their professional standards.

Recommendations

For this particular case, the art therapist recommended that all three siblings be placed in the same foster home in order to maintain a semblance of family unity. However, therapeutic considerations were overridden by social services, and the girls were separated. The therapist also recommended outpatient art therapy as a follow-up to treatment. This decision also was disregarded. As mentioned before, a case of this nature requires that therapists consult with each of the entities involved in the decision making process.

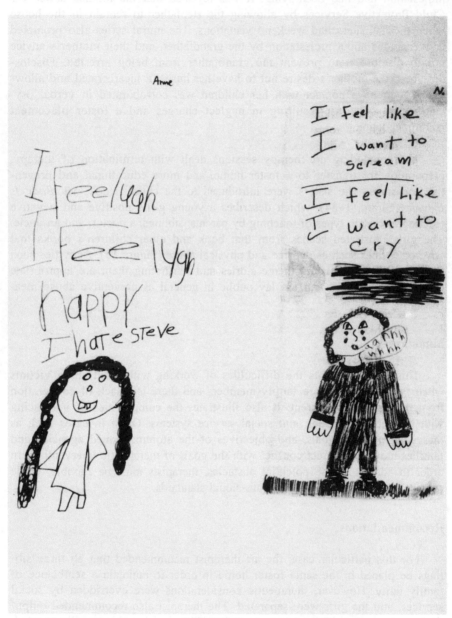

Figure 13. Anne and Nancy: "Feelings" (8" × 14½").

QUESTIONS

1. Discuss the implications of inpatient treatment for physical and sexual abuse cases involving children.
2. To what extent do outside agencies and organizations affect the treatment plan?
3. What is the relationship between actual sexual abuse and perceived sexual abuse in children's drawings?
4. What are some art activities appropriate for both diagnosis and treatment of child physical and sexual abuse victims?
5. In what ways can abuse interfere with victims' school performance?

REFERENCES

American Psychiatric Association. (1994). *Diagnostic and statistical manual of mental disorders* (fourth edition). Washington, DC: Author.

Dufrene, P. (1988). *A comparison of the traditional education of Native American healers with the education of American art therapists.* Ann Arbor, MI: University Microfilms International.

Girard, L. (1984). *My body is private.* Niles, IL: Whitman & Co.

Hagood, M. (1991). Group art therapy with mothers of sexually abused children. *The Arts in Psychotherapy, 18,* 17–27.

Manning, R. (1987). Aggression depicted in abused children's drawings. *The Arts in Psychotherapy, 14,* 15–24.

Powell, L. (1990). Treating sexually abused latency age girls. *The Arts in Psychotherapy, 17,* 35–47.

Serrano, J. (1989). The arts in therapy with survivors of incest. In H. Wadeson (Ed.), *Advances in art therapy* (pp. 114-125). New York: Wiley and Sons.

Sidun, N. (1987). Graphic indicators of sexual abuse in draw-a-person tests of psychiatrically hospitalized adolescents. *The Arts in Psychotherapy, 14,* 25–40.

Chapter 5

CASE STUDIES: FAMILIES

The authors have worked individually and as cotherapists on many family cases. The art therapy/psychotherapy treatments of two families (Case Studies 1–4 and Case Studies 5–8) are outlined in this chapter. In order to protect clients' identities, certain details have been changed.

CASE STUDY #1

In Case Studies 1–4, Coleman and Farris-Dufrene provided services to a dysfunctional family that had been involved with the juvenile and adult judicial system and the state welfare department. This family was referred to the authors by the family minister, their caseworker, and the superior court. The family included the mother, her live-in boyfriend, and her son and daughter. Case Studies 1–4 will focus on treatment for the entire family.

Brief Historical Overview

This case involves an African American male, Donald, 11 years old. Donald was molested by his paternal grandfather for three years while he resided with his grandparents. This sexual abuse resulted in Donald suffering from gender identity issues, conflict with his mother and sister, and difficulty with authority. As a ward of the state and former foster child, he is now reunited with his mother and receiving court mandated counseling from a multicultural therapeutic team consisting of a psychotherapist, art therapist, clinical social worker, and pastoral counselor.

Mental Status Evaluation

Donald is oriented to the three spheres of person, time, and place, and exhibited broad affect. He is extremely intelligent and articulate with an IQ of 135. He is above grade level on state standardized tests in mathematics and reading comprehension. Although Donald has been classified as gifted, due to his traumatic childhood, he exhibited inappropriate behaviors in academic, social, and family environments.

Empirical Observations

Assessed Psychological Impairment. Attempts were made by the multicultural treatment team to administer several psychological assessment tools. Donald's previous treatment history was such that he had experienced racial and cultural discrimination by therapists, physicians, the juvenile judicial system, and school personnel. Therefore, he refused to take what he perceived to be culturally biased instruments, and he did not want to risk being inaccurately labelled.

Disability Due to Impairment. Although Donald was 11 years old, he appeared to be much younger with respect to his size, and he periodically exhibited effeminate mannerisms, including wearing makeup and female clothing. These effeminate behaviors elicited confrontations with school faculty, staff, and students, often resulting in verbal and physical altercations. These altercations impaired his academic performance and social adjustment.

Diagnosis (Per the DSM-IV)

Donald

Axis I—Posttraumatic Stress Disorder, 309.81
  Adjustment Disorder with Depressed Mood, 309.00
  Parent–child Relational Problems, V61.20
Axis II—799.99, Diagnosis Deferred
Axis III—Calcaneal Spur
Axis IV—Psychosocial and Environmental Problems: Sexual Abuse, Separation Anxiety, Parent–child Relational Problems, Social Identity Issues
  Severity: Moderate to Severe
Axis V—Current GAF: 55
  Highest GAF Past Year: 55
  Previous GAF Prior to Counseling: 50 (serious symptoms, impairment in impulse control)

Systems Impact

Due to the severe impairment in Donald's functioning, there is a deleterious effect on his psychological, familial, academic, and social adjustment. Donald and his mother, sister, grandparents, and other relatives expressed apprehension related to the outcome of treatment and the final disposition of this case.

Treatment Plan

Treatment Modalities. Individual and family art and psychotherapy have been provided on a weekly basis for the past year. The authors will summarize the ongoing treatment process.

Introduction. Due to the complexities of Donald's situation, it initially was determined that a multicultural team approach would be more feasible in addressing his issues and concerns. Upon returning home from an unsatisfactory foster placement with a Caucasian lesbian couple, the court mandated the above treatment modality.

Initial Sessions. Farris-Dufrene met with Donald on several occasions at her office, his home, and his special education school. During these sessions, Donald utilized art therapy to portray graphically his feelings and concerns. With self-portraits, family portraits, and scenes from his school setting, Donald expressed his major emotional issues.

During a session in which Donald drew a family portrait, he illustrated a female figure on the left side of the page (Figure 14). This figure had a black bouffant hair style, large round face, green eyes, and large full mouth, was wearing an evening gown, and was holding a bouquet of flowers. Above the female's head, the word "LIFE" was written three times. Donald described this figure as his mother. A figure in the middle, identified as Donald himself, had a round face, green and black hair, stick lines for a neck, and outstretched arms and legs spread apart, and was dressed in black. On the right side he drew his sister, Carol, with long black hair, a smiling mouth, and a multicolored dress shaped like a valentine. In the top right corner of the page, Donald drew a large round shaped figure with legs and arms in profile, a tiny head, and curly hair. This person was unidentified. None of the three major figures had any interaction with each other. Of all of the three figures, Donald deemphasized himself the most.

Additional Sessions. In subsequent art therapy sessions, Donald was reluctant to portray visually scenes from his school environment, such as field trips,

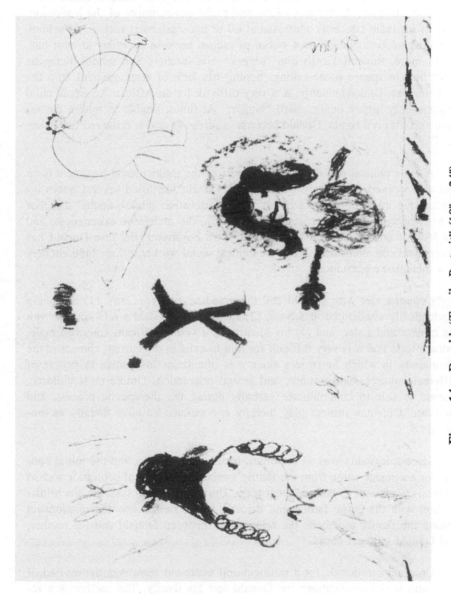

Figure 14. Donald: "Family Portrait" (18" × 24").

other classmates, and school activities. His refusal to draw school related activities was attributed to the insensitive and racist environment of the institution. One of his main concerns addressed at all of his sessions is racism. At school, Donald perceives himself as a victim of racism because everyday at least one, if not more, student(s) calls him "nigger." His teachers and school therapists want him to ignore name-calling, hoping his lack of response will stop the verbal abuse. Understandably, it is very difficult for an African American child to constantly ignore being called "nigger." At times, unable to ignore the assaults on his civil rights, Donald becomes aggressive and is removed for "time-out."

A male clinical social worker was part of the multicultural treatment team and also worked extensively with Donald. Donald identified several issues including the inappropriateness of his special education school, adults' disbelief in his responses to their constant interrogation, the racism he experiences, and his lack of communication with his mother's boyfriend. Because Donald has exceptional communication skills, the clinical social worker utilizes bibliotherapy as a therapeutic technique.

Coleman met with Donald and discussed several concerns: (1) not being academically challenged at school, (2) racism, (3) Donald's relationship with his mother and sister, and (4) his identity as a young African American male. Donald feels that it is very difficult for him to exist in the current climate in the community in which he resides since it is oftentimes insensitive to people of different cultures, backgrounds, and sexual orientation. Unlike most children, Donald is able to communicate verbally during the therapeutic process, and therefore, Coleman utilizes play therapy and rational emotive therapy as modalities.

Since spirituality was an important focus of the family, and the initial contact for assistance came from the family's minister, a pastoral counselor was an integral component of the treatment team. During the initial sessions, the minister met with the entire family and discussed their new home, the relationship among the family members, the relationship between Donald and his mother, and Donald's sexual abuse.

One major rationale for a multicultural treatment team was the myriad of legal and social implications for Donald and his family. The mother is a recovering alcoholic and substance abuser, currently living with a Caucasian man who frequently physically and psychologically abuses her. Law enforcement officials have intervened on many occasions. Unfortunately, Donald has been involved in verbal and physical altercations with the live-in boyfriend in an attempt to protect and defend his mother. This has resulted in ongoing legal discussions concerning the efficacy of Donald remaining at home with his mother or being removed to another foster home or institutionalization. All of these external factors have been obstacles to the therapeutic process, as the treatment team has been required to respond to each crisis.

Towards the conclusion of the academic year, Farris-Dufrene met with Donald several times in the school setting. Donald requested that he be provided textbooks and supplementary materials more appropriate for his reading level. He was cooperative in wanting to express his feelings via art therapy. During a session at the end of the spring semester, Donald used pastels to draw a large flower dominating the paper (Figure 15). A blue sky was drawn across the top of the page, along with a yellow sun with rays in the corner. The flower had purple petals, a white center, and a yellow circle in the middle. It is almost as tall as the sun and sky. A green stem, leaves, and brown roots were drawn under the light green grass. This pretty, decorative image may be interpreted as a denial of Donald's true feelings and issues. It is his way of trying to cover up negative issues he does not want to discuss. Also, it is a somewhat stereo-typically drawn image that could have been done by a younger child. Donald was hesitant to leave the art therapy session and return to the classroom. This was a reflection of him being uncomfortable in the special education academic setting.

Therapeutically, this case is significant in that it utilizes a multicultural, multidisciplinary treatment team that continues to work cooperatively in an effort to facilitate the adjustment of Donald and the other family members. This case was also unique because it was the first time that this type of treatment modality was approved and mandated by the juvenile justice system in the authors' state. As of the writing of this book, the treatment team is continuing to provide therapeutic intervention as needed for Donald, his sister (Carol), his mother, and her male companion.

CASE STUDY #2

Brief Historical Overview

This case involves Carol, a 17-year-old senior in high school in a small Midwestern community. She initially was included in counseling and psycho-therapy due to the court order for the entire Williams family to be treated. Carol has lived with various relatives, including her grandmother, aunt, and

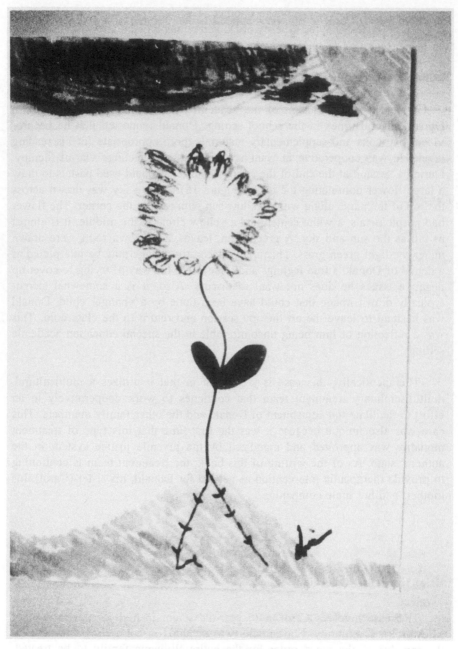

Figure 15.   Donald: "Flower" (8" × 10").

biological father. Due to being separated from her mother for many of her formative years, Carol is not very bonded to her mother and younger brother (Donald).

Mental Status Evaluation

Carol is oriented to the three spheres of person, time, and place, and is very articulate and well-groomed. The mental status evaluation indicated that she has excellent recent and remote memory, and her judgment is good. Her academic performance is at grade level, scoring average on standardized tests.

Empirical Observations

Assessed Psychological Impairment. Coleman did not administer any psychological assessments to Carol. During Carol's initial presentation, it was determined that these tools were unnecessary at the time.

Disability Due to Impairment. In the initial stages of therapy, Coleman and Farris-Dufrene did not observe any indications of disability. At that time, Carol was residing with her maternal grandmother and had minimal contact with her mother and brother. However, as she was required by the court to have more interaction with her mother and brother, her emotional and psychological state deteriorated. The attempted reunion with her mother and brother brought back painful repressed memories of family separation, domestic violence, and alcohol and substance abuse.

Diagnosis (Per the DSM-IV)

Carol

Axis I—Posttraumatic Stress Disorder, 309.81
   Eating Disorder, NOS, 307.50
   Academic Problem, V62.30
Axis II—799.90, Diagnosis Deferred
Axis III—Lumps in Breast, Undiagnosed Gynecological Problems
Axis IV—Psychosocial and Environmental Problems: Abandonment, Neglect
   Severity: Mild to Moderate
Axis V—Current GAF: 65 (mild to moderate)
   Highest GAF Past Year: 90 (absent)
   Previous GAF Prior to Counseling: 90

Systems Impact

Carol's attempts to reunite with her dysfunctional family adversely affected her academic performance, leading to several school suspensions. Her inappropriate behavior led to placement in a group home for girls.

Treatment Plan

Treatment Modalities. The treatment consisted of individual art therapy with Farris-Dufrene, coupled with family therapy provided by Coleman and academic tutoring at a local community center.

Introduction. The team of therapists decided that in order to facilitate positive growth, Carol also should participate in art therapy due to her interests in modeling, and interior and fashion design. It also was determined by the team that Carol needed a therapist who did not work individually with her mother, since the mother-daughter relationship was a primary issue.

Initial Session. Due to the mother's noncompliance with the therapeutic process in terms of transportation for her daughter, Farris-Dufrene had to meet with Carol at her home. The first session was two hours long, and art therapy was utilized to portray graphically Carol's issues concerning the school environment. She had been suspended twice during the semester and was worried about her educational future. Carol also was concerned about racism and discrimination at the predominantly white high school. She felt that although she was guilty of late arrivals and one incident of fighting, the punishment was too severe. Carol wanted to have therapeutic intervention at the high school instead of suspension/expulsion for her school infractions. She thought that she was being treated harshly because of her African American ancestry and attending school in a predominantly white environment.

In her family portrait, Carol drew 15 figures lined in a row, including cousins, grandparents, aunts, uncles, and her father, mother, and brother (Figure 16). All of the figures were drawn in brown pencil with round faces, no necks, arms pressed close to the sides and torsos and legs merging into one long rectangular shape. All of the people had similar facial features/expressions. A dollar sign was drawn next to the head of one uncle. There was no picture of Carol in the family portrait.

Because of Carol's exclusion of herself in the family portrait, the art therapist requested that she draw an individual self-portrait (Figure 17). Carol portrayed

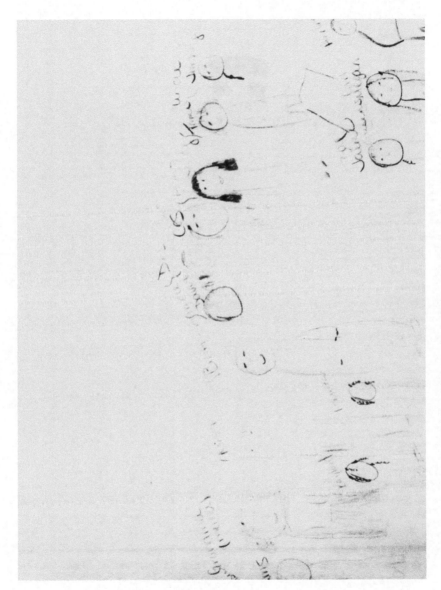

Figure 16. Carol: "Family Portrait" (18" × 24").

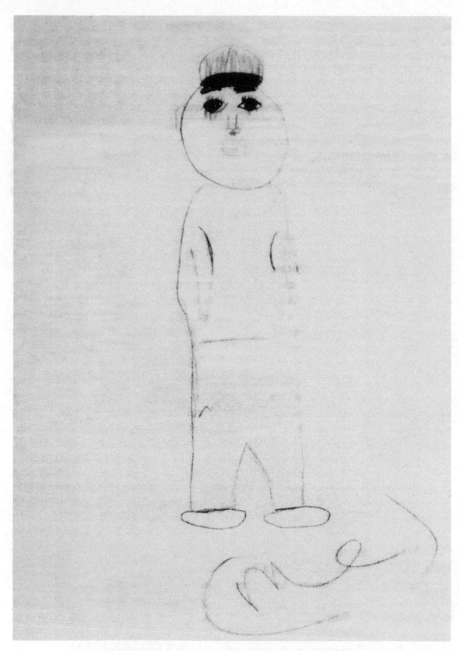

Figure 17.   Carol: "Self-portrait" (18" × 24").

herself as very tall, with a round face and no neck, large dark eyes and lashes, and short arms pressed to the sides of her chest. The figure appears to be wearing pants, but a wavy, horizontal line across the legs may indicate a dress or skirt. These drawings may suggest that Carol does not feel that she is part of the family system.

Farris-Dufrene identified several issues and concerns that Carol needed to address in therapy, including self-esteem, the racial harassment at the predominantly white high school, academic performance, and the relationship with her mother. The therapist was extremely concerned about the volatile racial environment at the high school and consulted with the principal about the incidents involving Carol—in particular, the incident where a student wrote "nigger" on Carol's locker.

Additional Sessions. Due to Mrs. Williams' further noncompliance, Farris-Dufrene was unable to meet formally with Carol for several months. However, Farris-Dufrene did communicate with Carol by telephone concerning her expulsion from the high school and a racially motivated incident related to verbal and physical altercations. As a result of the expulsion, Farris-Dufrene was invited to the high school for a meeting that included the principal, the guidance counselor, Carol, and her mother. Several options were discussed for resolving the personal and school conflict, but Mrs. Williams preferred institutionalization for her daughter. The principal and Farris-Dufrene did not agree with Mrs. Williams' recommendation; however, the parent had final authority and felt she could not handle her own issues and problems plus Carol and all of her issues and problems. At the time of this writing, Carol is residing in a group home for delinquent girls, much to the dismay of the entire treatment team.

CASE STUDY #3

Brief Historical Overview

This case involves Donald and Carol's mother, an African American female, Linda, age 42. Linda has a history of alcohol and substance abuse, and was previously in treatment. As a result of her alcoholism and substance abuse, she frequently has lost and regained custody of her two children, who usually were placed with their paternal grandparents.

Linda currently is living with a white male factory worker who also has a history of alcoholism and substance abuse. She has been involved in this relationship for three years. Law enforcement officials have been summoned on several occasions due to verbal and physical altercations between the two, and the relationship is quite tenuous, at best.

Mental Status Evaluation

Linda is oriented to the three spheres of person, time, and place, and exhibited broad affect. She is extremely articulate, well-groomed, assertive, and quite knowledgeable of the mental health and judicial systems. Linda has completed her GED and is currently a student in a hospital-based RN program, with plans to continue on for her bachelor's degree in nursing.

Empirical Observations

Assessed Psychological Impairment. Linda previously had been tested by psychologists during her treatment, and the reports indicated that her IQ was in the above average range; she did not exhibit any psychological disorders or impairment. She has been drug free for the past five years but continues to abuse alcohol frequently.

Disability Due to Impairment. Linda continues to abuse alcohol, having weekend binges that have an adverse impact on her educational goals and objectives, specifically, her ability to study and maintain a minimum grade point average. These binges oftentimes result in absenteeism, physical abuse, separations, and neglect of her children. However, during her separations from her boyfriend, Linda refrains from alcohol abuse and is capable of functioning on a day-to-day basis.

Diagnosis (Per the DSM-IV)

Linda

> Axis I—Alcohol Abuse, 305.00
> Adjustment Disorder with Depressed Mood, 309.00
> Parent–child Relational Problems, V61.20
> Axis II—799.90, Diagnosis Deferred
> Axis III—None
> Axis IV—Psychosocial and Environmental Problems: Alcohol Abuse, Parent–child Relational Problems, Physical Abuse, Financial Difficulties
> Severity: Moderate to Severe

Axis V—Current GAF: 60
   Highest GAF Past Year: 60
   Previous GAF Prior to Counseling: 50 (serious symptoms, impairment in alcohol abuse)

Systems Impact

The effect of the alcohol abuse, verbal and physical altercations, financial obligations, and parent–child conflict have caused Linda to develop inappropriate coping mechanisms, specifically with regard to her child-rearing. She appears to devote more energy to maintaining a dysfunctional relationship with her boyfriend than to focusing on improving the relationships with her adolescent daughter and son.

Treatment Plan

Treatment Modalities. Individual and family psychotherapy were provided several times each week in order to help Linda cope with her daily stressors. Linda was resistant to art therapy and also to the relationship that Farris-Dufrene established with Linda's daughter (Carol).

Introduction. Linda's treatment was another component of the multicultural team approach that had been designed for her children, Donald and Carol.

Initial Sessions. Coleman met with Linda initially to discuss the process and how the team would facilitate positive growth among the entire family. The focuses of these sessions were on increasing Linda's self-esteem, helping her develop more appropriate defense mechanisms, and teaching new strategies and techniques for parenting. Linda had not developed a positive relationship with her mother, and this emotional strain oftentimes was manifested in the relationship with Linda's two children, especially her daughter, Carol.

The recommendation for Linda also to meet with Farris-Dufrene for art therapy was not accepted by Linda. Linda felt that Farris-Dufrene did not support her efforts to parent and discipline Carol, and disagreed with Farris-Dufrene's assessment that Linda favored Donald over Carol.

Additional Sessions. Subsequent psychotherapy sessions with Coleman dealt more in-depth with attempting to help Linda identify issues related to her self-worth, how to cope with the alcohol abuse, and the impaired relationship with her boyfriend. Linda also spent a significant amount of time trying to understand how she could continue to stay in a relationship that was verbally and physically abusive. This relationship, particularly the physical abuse, was the cause, in one incident, of her son being placed in a mental health institution for long-term care.

Due to Linda's above average intelligence, she was quite able to articulate her feelings of insecurity and low self-esteem. She fully understood the dynamics of her situation, even though in most instances she was unable to progress psychologically enough to implement change in her life.

While Donald was institutionalized, Linda was not compliant with treatment, continued to abuse alcohol, continued to neglect her daughter's physical and mental health, and sustained verbal and physical abuse from her live-in lover, Dick. This type of behavior was present at the time of the completion of this book.

CASE STUDY #4

Brief Historical Overview

This case involves a 43-year-old Caucasian male, Dick, who has resided with Linda and her two children, Carol and Donald, for three years. Dick is a blue-collar worker in a local factory, having been employed immediately upon dropping out of high school. He has a history of alcoholism and substance abuse. Dick presented as unkempt and not caring about his personal grooming or appearance.

Mental Status Evaluation

Dick is oriented to the three spheres of person, time, and place, and exhibited flat affect. He is of average intelligence, and while he may have average verbal skills, most of the time he is reticent and unable to express or articulate his feelings or thoughts.

Empirical Observations

Assessed Psychological Impairment. Dick was quite resistant to treatment and would not participate in any psychological assessment procedures. He was apprehensive about the counseling and psychotherapeutic process, having been reared by a Pentecostal minister (who did not believe in "nontraditional" treatments such as counseling) and homemaker, and having not participated previously in counseling.

Disability Due to Impairment. Because of Dick's lack of formal education or job training, as well as a history of alcohol abuse, he is unable to acquire employment that would allow him to support Linda and her two children. While he is able to function at work, he continues to abuse alcohol during the evenings and on weekends.

Diagnosis (Per the DSM-IV)

<u>Dick</u>

Axis I—Alcohol Abuse, 305.00
Adjustment Disorder with Depressed Mood, 309.00
Partner Relational Problem, V61.10
Axis II—799.90, Diagnosis Deferred
Axis III—Unknown
Axis IV—Psychosocial and Environmental Problems: Alcohol Abuse, Physical Abuse, Financial Difficulties
Severity: Moderate to Severe
Axis V—Current GAF: 55
Highest GAF Past Year: 55
Previous GAF Prior to Counseling: 50 (serious symptoms, impairment in alcohol abuse)

Systems Impact

Dick's abuse of alcohol, the frequent verbal and physical altercations with Linda, and the financial strain and obligations resulted in severe impairment in the relationship. While there were several breakups during the relationship, there appeared to be no commitment from Dick to identifying his issues and concerns and working on improving the relationship with Linda and her children. The relationship with Donald was especially impaired, as Donald had observed, on several occasions, Dick physically assaulting Donald's mother. During the most recent physical altercation, Donald had intervened in order to protect Linda, and she still sustained a black eye and other bruises and abrasions.

Treatment Plan

Treatment Modalities. The treatment team met with the family, including Dick, on five occasions, and Coleman attempted individual counseling and psychotherapy. Dick was not receptive to treatment or the therapeutic process, and although he would attend sessions, he did not speak most of the time or address any of his concerns.

Introduction. The individual sessions were utilized to help Dick understand the purpose of counseling and how it would facilitate a better relationship and interaction between and among Linda, Carol, and Donald. Since Dick did not see the significance of counseling, he did not believe that it would help the situation. Initially, he agreed to cooperate; however, he oftentimes was late for appointments or cancelled the sessions.

Sessions. Coleman spent the initial sessions outlining the family dynamics and the importance of Dick participating in the therapeutic process. Although Dick appeared to understand and comply with treatment, as the verbal and physical altercations with Linda escalated he began to retreat into his own fantasy world, denying that problems existed. As the situation with Linda deteriorated, so did Dick's interaction with Donald. Dick felt that Donald, due to his special needs, required too much of Linda's attention. Dick's pathology prevented him from acknowledging his own needs, resulting in a more impaired triangular relationship with Linda and the children.

RECOMMENDATIONS FOR CASES 1–4

The authors suggest that for this highly dysfunctional family, individual and family therapy will be a lifelong process. The treatment team, including the outside agencies and judicial system, is highly critical of the living arrangement between the mother and her boyfriend due to his alcoholism and physical abuse. It is felt that his presence in the home is detrimental to the healthy psychosocial development of the children. It also was determined that he was a codependent in the relationship with the mother, and therefore prohibited her from developing her full potential professionally and socially. Another recommendation is the transfer of Donald to a another educational institution that is more receptive to the issues, needs, and concerns of multicultural and diverse populations.

A decision that created much controversy between the treatment team and the various agencies was the institutionalization of Donald. While the treatment team was not against institutionalization theoretically, it felt that there were no appropriate facilities within the state that could accommodate children who had similar experiences to Donald's.

Cases 1–4 together are an example of a multidisciplinary treatment approach to family therapy. These cases highlight various levels of authority and decision making, and the necessity for all parties to communicate and cooperate for the general welfare of the clients.

QUESTIONS FOR CASES 1–4

1. How would one outline the various issues that Donald experienced upon referral to treatment?
2. What is Carol's position within the family system? How does her position impact the family dynamics?
3. How might a therapist deal with the denial and resistance in a client such as Linda?
4. In what ways do alcoholism and physical abuse influence the male/female relationship?
5. What are the benefits of the use and nonuse of art therapy within this particular family?

CASE STUDY #5

In Case Studies 5–8, the authors provided art therapy and psychotherapy services to an economically disadvantaged Caucasian family who received financial support from the state department of welfare. This family was referred to the authors by their pastoral counselor. This is a blended family that includes a recently married husband and wife, Henry and Diane. Henry's children are a 15-year-old daughter, Cathy; a 17-year-old son, John; and a 12-year-old son, Ronald. Diane's children include Betty, a 5-year-old, and a 1-year-old biracial daughter, LaKisha, by an African American father.

This family presented with a complexity of issues and concerns that resulted in multiple diagnoses for each member. The authors will focus first on the husband, Henry (Case Study #5), followed by Diane (Case Study #6), and then the children (Case Study #7 and Case Study #8).

Brief Historical Overview

Henry is an unskilled, unemployed, middle-aged man who has been on public assistance for most of his adult life. His infrequent attempts at employment included a brief stints in the United States Army National Guard and as a hospital orderly. He is divorced from the mother of his children, a chronic alcoholic judged unfit for parenting by the state. After a very short courtship (less than one month), Henry married a welfare dependent mother who had one child and who was also 7 months pregnant by an African American male. Henry has been in treatment for several years for various situations/issues.

Mental Status Evaluation

Henry is oriented to the three spheres of person, time, and space, and exhibited a labile affect. His IQ is borderline/normal (95). Henry presented with several of the criteria identified for Histrionic Personality Disorder. For example, he often pretended to be a physician, even convincing his biological and stepchildren of such. Henry frequently displayed inappropriate affection toward the therapists and other females. What was disconcerting to the treatment team was Henry's lack of attention to his personal hygiene; the stench, at times, was overwhelming. The entire family displayed poor personal and home hygiene.

Empirical Observations

Assessed Psychological Impairment. Several attempts were made by the authors to administer IQ, projective, and personality inventories. However, Henry was not amenable to these requests. He believed that because he had been employed briefly in a medical environment as an orderly, he was too advanced to be measured by traditional psychological evaluation. The authors, therefore, had to refer to previously conducted psychological evaluations.

Disability Due to Impairment. Although Henry is physically able to work, he resists vocational counseling and employment. Henry made frequent requests of the authors to provide written documentation that he was physically and mentally incapable of performing minimum duties. At this stage of his life, Henry was totally welfare dependent, a behavior and attitude that affected his wife and children.

Diagnosis (Per the DSM-IV)

<u>Henry</u>

Axis I—Partner Relational Problem, V61.1
Parent–child Conflict, V61.20
Axis II—Histrionic Personality Disorder, 301.50

Axis III—None Presented
Axis IV—Psychosocial and Environmental Problems: Occupational, Relational, Economic, and Psychological
Axis V—Current GAF: 40
    Highest GAF Past Year: 50
    Previous GAF Prior to Counseling: 40

Systems Impact

Due to Henry's severe impairment in his functioning, there is a deleterious effect on his psychological, familial, occupational, and social adjustment. As head of the household, Henry established an environment that promulgated a cycle of dependency.

CASE STUDY #6

Brief Historical Overview

Diane is a 30-year-old Caucasian female from Appalachia who recently migrated to the Midwest. She recently divorced her first husband who had physically assaulted her and sexually assaulted their daughter. Shortly after the divorce, Diane became pregnant by an African American man. Her current husband, Henry, has adopted the biracial daughter. Diane did not complete high school and has never been employed.

Mental Status Evaluation

Diane is oriented to the three spheres of person, time, and place. She presented with a flat affect, and she has a borderline IQ of 90. Diane is suffering from Dysthymic Disorder and has very low self-esteem. Because of the severity of her depression, she currently is being treated with Prozac.

Empirical Observations

Assessed Psychological Impairment. The authors determined that due to Diane's low self-esteem, it was inappropriate to administer psychological instruments at this time. Medical and psychological records from previous clinicians were analyzed; their conclusions supported this decision.

Disability Due to Impairment. Diane's lack of energy, poor concentration, and insomnia interfered with her ability to pursue a GED and employment. Like her husband, Henry, Diane also exhibited poor personal and family hygiene habits. The family clothing, home, and environment were substandard, prompting an investigation by the state welfare department. The authors encouraged Diane to enroll in a publicly-funded homemaking class. Although she enrolled, she was not compliant. Additional complaints came from school authorities specifically concerning the children's unkempt, unsanitary, unhygienic appearance and their seeming lack of proper nutrition.

Diagnosis (Per the DSM-IV)

Diane

Axis I—Partner Relational Problem, V61.1
Parent–child Conflict, V61.20
Axis II—799.99, Diagnosis Deferred
Axis III—None Presented
Axis IV—Psychosocial and Environmental Problems: Occupational, Relational, Economic, and Psychological
Axis V—Current GAF: 40
Highest GAF Past Year: 45
Previous GAF Prior to Counseling: 40

Systems Impact

Diane's impairment in her functioning resulted in a deleterious effect on her psychological, occupational, social, and familial adjustment. As a mother, she neglected her children and was unable to provide their basic physiological and safety needs.

CASE STUDY #7

Brief Historical Overview

Cathy is a 15-year-old Caucasian female with a learning disability, auditory hallucinations, and various physical problems (irritable bowel syndrome, external otitis, and migraine headaches). She is enrolled in special education at the local high school and is under medication management for her psychological issues.

Mental Status Evaluation

Cathy is oriented to the three spheres of person, time, and place, with a broad affect. Her IQ is in the normal range. Having been sexually assaulted at age 4, she expressed suicidal ideations and claustrophobia. Cathy is immature and too demanding of attention.

Empirical Observations

Assessed Psychological Impairment. Since Cathy was enrolled in special education classes, psychological testing was provided by the school system. Although learning disabled, she is an avid reader and also keeps a diary.

Disability Due to Impairment. Due to her aforementioned physical and psychological problems, Cathy is frequently absent from school and, therefore, behind in her academic work. At times, home tutoring has been provided. Cathy has no close friends at school or in the neighborhood, possibly due to her inappropriate behaviors.

Diagnosis (Per the DSM-IV)

Cathy

Axis I—Posttraumatic Stress Disorder, 309.81
    Parent–child Conflict, V61.20
Axis II—799.99, Diagnosis Deferred
Axis III—Irritable Bowel Syndrome, External Otitis, Migraine Headaches
Axis IV—Psychosocial and Environmental Problems: Academic, Relational, and Psychological
Axis V—Current GAF: 55
    Highest GAF Past Year: 50
    Previous GAF Prior to Counseling: 55

Systems Impact

Due to Cathy's learning disability and physiological problems, there is a deleterious effect on her academic, social, psychological, and familial functioning.

CASE STUDY #8

Brief Historical Overview

John is a 17-year-old Caucasian male who was involved in the juvenile justice system, having been caught shoplifting, defacing property, and being truant. He prefers to devote most of his time socializing with his peer group, members of a teenage gang.

Mental Status Evaluation

John is oriented to the three spheres of person, time, and place, with a broad affect. His IQ is 110, and school officials suggested that he has the ability to perform above average academically.

Empirical Observations

Assessed Psychological Impairment. John was rebellious and resisted the idea of seeing therapists because he was "not crazy." He previously was diagnosed as having a Conduct Disorder.

Diagnosis (Per the DSM-IV)

John

Axis I—Posttraumatic Stress Disorder, 309.81
     Parent–child Conflict, V61.20
Axis II—799.99, Diagnosis Deferred
Axis III—None Presented
Axis IV—Psychosocial and Environment Problems: Academic, Relational, and Psychological
Axis V—Current GAF: 55
     Highest GAF Past Year: 50
     Previous GAF Prior to Counseling: 50

Systems Impact

Due to John's academic and psychological impairment, his functioning at school and at home was inappropriate and immature. As the oldest child, he was not a positive role model for the other children.

Treatment Plan

Treatment Modalities. The treatment consisted of family psychotherapy with Coleman, coupled with individual art therapy for Cathy and John.

Introduction. While the family initially presented to Coleman, she determined that it would be appropriate to invite Farris-Dufrene as cotherapist in order to provide art therapy for the children. Treatment for the family has continued, despite more economic, social, and psychological hardship. Although the family is supported by the state department of welfare, the therapists were unable to be fully reimbursed for their services.

Initial Session. During the initial session, the entire blended family presented. Each member was dirty and had an unpleasant odor. There was constant bickering among the children, and the parents did not possess the skills for intervention or disciplining the children. Each child was competing for attention from his or her respective biological parent. Another issue of concern was how the children should refer to their stepparents. Although both parents wanted to be called "mom and dad," the children wanted to call the step-parent by his or her first name. It took quite a while for the therapists to initiate a behavior management plan for the therapy sessions.

The therapists outlined specific treatment goals for the family as a whole and individually. Henry's primary goal was to seek vocational training and/or employment. Diane's focus was on developing appropriate parenting and home-making skills through available community resources. The goal for John was to adhere to the guidelines established by his probation officer, especially improving attendance at school. Because of Cathy's severe medical problems, the therapists emphasized the importance of compliance with medication instructions. In conjunction with school officials, the team agreed to monitor Cathy's behavior with respect to medication. Twelve-year-old Ronald, who is extremely quiet and withdrawn, has the goal of learning to be more assertive within the family system. Betty, the 5-year-old and a victim of sexual assault, displays inappropriate behavior in public, such as masturbation. The therapists decided that her goals should be to understand the sexual assault and develop mechanisms for informing her mother or other adults if similar situations occur in the future. A goal for the family with respect to LaKisha, the biracial daughter, was to provide Afro-centric experiences for her as she gets older. In compliance with this, the family joined a multicultural church.

Additional Sessions. Farris-Dufrene met with John and Cathy for individual art therapy. During one of the initial sessions, John drew two homes.

The first house that he drew is tilted on the ground and surrounded by a barren background (Figure 18). The front of the house is partly bricked, with a domed-shaped doorway that resembles a fireplace or oven. He did not draw any windows or chimney. The roof is black. Next to the house is a tree, uncolored. To illustrate the leaves, John drew a circular shape, similar to the schema drawn by elementary children. On the whole, the drawing appears to be that of a much younger person. John did not wish to add any other physical features to the house or any other people to his drawing. This drawing was executed when he was in a somewhat depressed mood.

In a subsequent individual art therapy session, John drew a house that was more age appropriate (Figure 19). Using pastel colored chalk, John drew a sky background using an intense blue. The roof of the house was colored black, the upper level of the house was magenta, and the lower level was grey. A magenta door was framed by a black border. Using heavy hand pressure, John made all of the colors intense. The room in one window appears to have a light on, and the other window is darkened. This drawing is much stronger, more forceful, and moodier than the other drawings. It illustrates more maturity and age appropriate drawing skills.

The first house seemed to indicate that John perceived his home as not having a firm foundation or structure. This may indicate the uncertainty surrounding the remarriage of his father and accepting step-siblings. John's desire to leave the drawing partially incomplete and barren suggests that John felt his current home environment was empty and meaningless. Although the second drawing is somewhat moody, with suggestions of depression, it does exhibit some strengths. For example, unlike the first house, this house has windows with a light on and is multicolored, and the drawing and background fill the entire sheet of paper. The light may indicate family interaction and hope for a brighter future.

During art therapy sessions, Cathy focused on drawing family members. Her first drawing was entitled "Old Family" (Figure 20). It consisted of her nuclear family prior to her biological parents' divorce and her father's remarriage. The people are drawn in childish, stick figure schemas. The family is enclosed in a frame. Although the biological mother is drawn larger, often indicating importance, during conversations about the family, the mother is seldom mentioned by Cathy or the other children.

In a subsequent session, Cathy drew a picture entitled "New Family" (Figure 21). The figures mainly consist of round faces that represent the whole

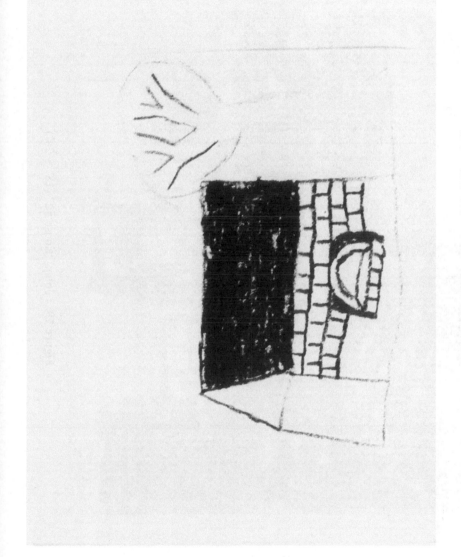

Figure 18. John: "House #1" (18" × 24").

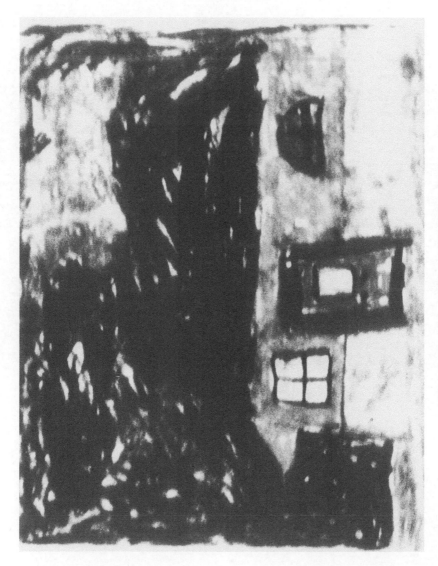

Figure 19. John: "House #2" (18" × 24").

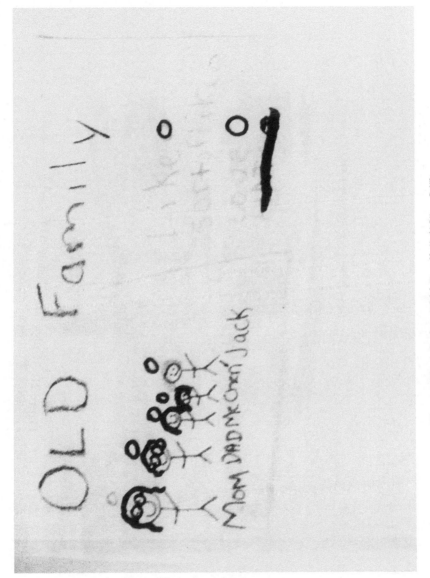

Figure 20. Cathy: "Old Family" (18" × 24").

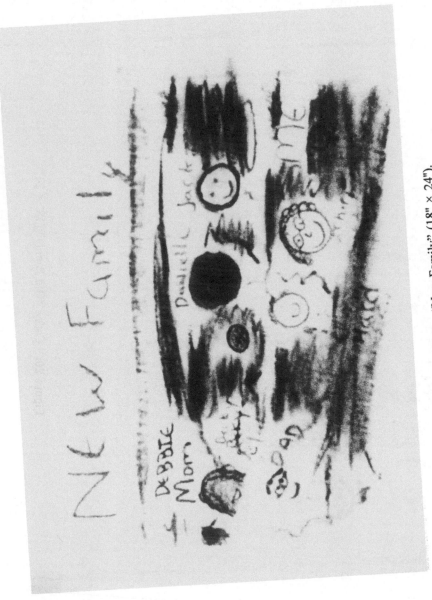

Figure 21. Cathy: "New Family" (18" × 24").

body, with small appendages for arms and legs. In the left-hand corner is the mother's name and the word "Mom" below it. These two words represent Cathy's conflict over whether to call the stepmother by her first name or "Mom." The stepmother prefers to be called "Mom," but Cathy insists on calling the stepmother by her first name. This is a continuing source of conflict between stepmother and stepdaughter.

Another family portrait has people portrayed as stick figures (Figure 22). The figures have no facial features, no clothing, and no gender differentiation. Their names are written above their heads. In this scene, the family members are not interacting with each other and are not surrounded by any type of environment.

This series of drawings focuses on the major family issues for Cathy, such as her father's remarriage, her acceptance/nonacceptance of step-siblings, and her position in the new family. Although she is in high school, the drawings appear to be those of a much younger child. Even though Cathy is enrolled in special education classes, her cognitive skills indicated that she could draw on a more age appropriate level. Since these are major individual and family issues, it is critical that treatment be continued on a long-term basis, utilizing art therapy and psychotherapy.

RECOMMENDATIONS FOR CASES 5–8

The authors believe that this extremely dysfunctional family will require individual and family therapy over an extended period of time. The therapists, including outside institutions such as the public school and the judicial system, are highly critical of the father's refusal to work and both parents' lack of parenting and homemaking skills. It is felt that the current state of the home creates psychological stressors and is, therefore, detrimental to the welfare of the family and children.

QUESTIONS FOR CASES 5–8

1. How would one outline the various issues that family members experienced upon referral to treatment?
2. With Henry as the head of household, what implications did his unemployment have on the family dynamics?
3. How might Diane facilitate the step-siblings accepting each other?

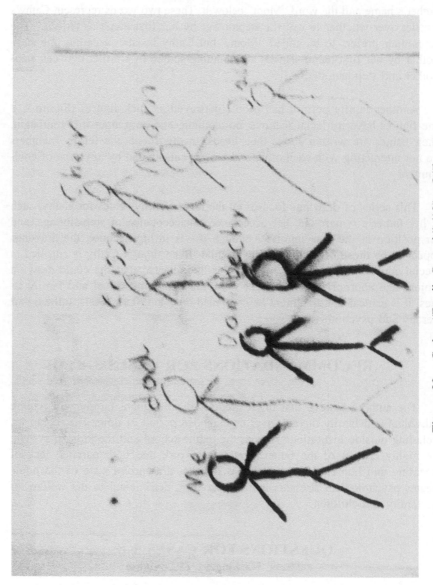

Figure 22. Cathy: "Family Portrait" (18" × 24").

4. What strategies might be helpful for this blended family to become more unified?
5. What were the benefits of the use of art therapy with the two adolescents?

SUMMARY OF INDIVIDUAL AND FAMILY SESSIONS

The aforementioned discussions of psychotherapy and art therapy illustrate the necessities and complexities of providing mental health services for families. Utilizing the systems approach, the authors identified issues and concerns of each individual family member and possible treatment modalities to address these concerns. The family dynamics should indicate how one modality may be preferable over another depending on the personality characteristics of each respective family member. The success of family therapy is contingent upon the careful assessment and analysis of each participant in the system, and his or her perception of counseling and the therapeutic process.

These cases are examples of a multidisciplinary treatment approach to family therapy. They highlight various levels of authority and decision making, and the necessity for all parties to communicate and cooperate for the general welfare of the clients.

The multicultural, multidisciplinary team concept was a dimension that was instrumental in facilitating the outcome of treatment in the aforementioned cases. The significance of cooperative efforts among service providers and the judicial and welfare systems further illustrates the future roles and responsibilities of mental health professionals. The authors continue to provide art therapy and psychotherapy for these families, often traveling to various institutions in order to service the children.

REFERENCE

American Psychiatric Association. (1994). *Diagnostic and statistical manual of mental disorders* (fourth edition). Washington, DC: Author.

Chapter **6**

CASE STUDIES: ADULTS

The authors have worked individually and as cotherapists on a number of cases involving adults. In this chapter are outlined three adult case studies and how the therapists used art therapy and psychotherapy to facilitate growth. In order to protect clients' identities, certain details have been changed.

CASE STUDY #1

Brief Historical Overview

This case involves Maryum, a Middle Eastern woman, age 45, who is married and has two sons. She has been under the care of Coleman since 1989. Maryum is suffering from Posttraumatic Stress Disorder and Depression resulting from sexual assault by a white male. Since that time, during treatment, Maryum has experienced extreme trauma resulting in depression, anxiety, fear, paranoia, and a series of stress related illnesses (i.e., insomnia, increases in appetite, heart palpitation, headaches, pain in various parts of the body, lack of interest in sex, and antisocial behavior). This incident has caused her to avoid contact with the outside world, and she does not participate as she previously did in everyday activities.

Mental Status Evaluation

The patient is oriented to the three spheres, with an affect that fluctuates from flat to labile. She is extremely intelligent and articulate. Maryum fre-

81

quently indicates several physiological concerns, specifically heart palpitation, numbness in both arms, headaches, insomnia, pain in various parts of the body, and lack of interest in sex. She also complains of not having much energy and of a poor appetite and eating habits. Her memory is fair, and her concentration will vary from poor to fair depending upon the circumstances. She did not present with delusional thinking or hallucinations.

Empirical Observations

Assessed Psychological Impairment. Clinical assessment and evaluation revealed that Maryum probably would meet the criteria for Posttraumatic Stress Disorder and Depression as delineated in the DSM-IV. Her situation is exacerbated by several psychosocial stressors including managing a home and assuming the roles of wife and mother of two children. She frequently has difficulty coping with these responsibilities, and her defense mechanisms are sometimes inappropriate.

Disability Due to Impairment. Professional observations and those of family members indicate that the client is having extreme difficulty readjusting to everyday life; consequently, there is major impairment in social, vocational, and other areas of her life. She often is involved in conflicts with her husband and children as a result of her mood, and she is frequently unable to handle these situations as she did before the incident. In this psychological and physiological condition, it has been extremely difficult for her to return to work. Due to the fact that she is having difficulty in the workplace, there has been a major financial adjustment for the family. She spends most of her time at home doing nothing and not participating in family activities. Consequently, her husband and children are having trouble adjusting to her behavior. Her husband, because of their religious background (Islamic), cannot accept the fact that she was violated sexually by a European American man.

Diagnosis (Per the DSM-IV)

Maryum

Axis I—Depressive Disorder, 311. 00
    Posttraumatic Stress Disorder, 309. 81
Axis II—799. 99, Diagnosis Deferred
Axis III—Headaches, Insomnia, Various Pain, Heart Palpitation, Stomach Disorders, Fluctuations in Appetite and Weight
Axis IV—Psychosocial and Environmental Problems: Anxiety, Depression,

Physical Ailments, Social Impairment, Decrease in Financial Status, Conflict with Children
    Severity: Extreme
Axis V—Current GAF: 40
    Highest GAF Past Year: 40
    Previous GAF Prior to Assault: 90

Systems Impact

Because Maryum is not able to function as she did prior to the assault, this has had a deleterious effect on her as an individual and also on her family life. Relations with her husband and children have seriously deteriorated, as she is unable to perform as she did prior to 1986 (time of assault). Consequently, her husband, children, family, friends, and others have been affected by the sexual assault.

Underlying Character and Value System

Before the sexual assault, Maryum was a dynamic, intelligent, articulate middle-aged professional who was able to assume many roles as mother, wife, and career woman. However, since the incident, she is anxious, paranoid, and suffers from depression. Her daily activities have been seriously impaired as a result of this experience.

Treatment Plan

Treatment Modalities. Individual and family psychotherapy, along with medication management, were provided on a weekly basis for one year. During the second year, art therapy consultations were provided as needed. The authors will summarize the treatment process through the time of the writing of this book.

Introduction. During the first year of individual and family psychotherapy, traditional "talk therapy" was sufficient enough to provide adequate therapeutic intervention. However, it became apparent that additional modalities and techniques were necessary to facilitate Maryum's healing process and readjustment.

Initial Session. The initial sessions focused on helping the client understand that it was not her fault that she was violated sexually. These sessions

IMPAIRMENT PROFILE

CATEGORY MENTAL STATUS	IMPAIRMENT DESCRIPTION	IMPAIRMENT CLASS
Intelligence	Above average	1
Thinking	Frustrated by assault; anxious	4
Perception	Normal/slight deficit	3
Judgment	Impaired	3
Affect	Flat/labile	4
Behavior	Impaired	3
Rehabilitation Potential	Fair/good	4

Degrees of Impairment: 1 = 00–05% Impairment; 2 = 10–20%; 3 = 25–50%; 4 = 55–75%.

also dealt with her husband's sexual rejection of her based upon his religious beliefs. The therapist's goals centered on helping to reunite the couple and family and assisting Maryum in rebuilding her self-esteem. Approximately one year was devoted to addressing these therapeutic issues.

Art therapy consultations were initiated during the second year of individual psychotherapy for Maryum. While Maryum was excited about the prospect of having another therapist and therapeutic intervention to facilitate her growth, upon commencement of sessions provided by the art therapist, she became quite apprehensive.

Maryum's first drawing was executed in the upper right-hand corner of the paper, leaving the rest of the large white paper unused. The drawing consisted of a central figure surrounded by six smaller ones. The central figure (self-identified as the client) has a stereotypical cartoon/childish face with three dots for the eyes and nose and one horizontal line for the mouth. The head is hairless and does not have ears. There is a long, thick neck and an egg-shaped torso. Attached to the torso are long arms extending to the ground without joints, hands, or fingers. The short legs are shaped in a similar fashion. Two of the surrounding figures are laying on the ground, and four are standing. They have the same stereotypical head with dots for the features. However, the surrounding figures have three sticks protruding from the head to represent legs and arms. The two lines/sticks on the sides seem to symbolize the arms, and the one center line represents the legs. Maryum stated that the other figures were family members, but she did not specify which members. The drawing is similar to the imagery of pre-school children just beginning to draw human figures.

Later images showed a marked improvement in the client's ability to depict graphically herself and others. She exhibited less reluctance in drawing and did not have to be prompted to express herself visually. In one of her later drawings, Maryum used brown pastel chalk to draw a central figure with large circles for eyes, one vertical line for the nose, and a larger circle to represent an open mouth. The figure (the client) has ears and short curly hair. The upper torso/neck is represented by a vertical rectangle. A wider, almost square-shaped rectangle represents the lower torso/hips. The two arms have wrists, hands, and fingers. The left wrist has a yellow bracelet. The legs and feet are pointed toward two figures, one to the left and one to the right. The figure on the right also is executed in brown pastel chalk. In this figure, the round head is larger than the rest of the body. There are two circles for eyes, a bent line for the nose, and two horizontal lines shaped like a "V" portraying an open mouth. The hair is curly, and there are no ears. The neck/upper torso is shaped like the central figure's with the same box-like shape for the lower body and legs/feet going toward the right. There are no arms/hands. The figure on the left is done in black pastel chalk. It has three lines to represent the eyes and nose and a circle to represent an open mouth. The figure has black curly hair and the same body type as the other two figures. The main difference is that the lower box-like torso is drawn over the legs. The legs show through the "skirt," and the feet protrude at the bottom. Both figures on the sides are smaller than the central figure.

The early drawings suggest that Maryum had very low self-esteem and perceived herself in a childlike manner. Her drawing ability had regressed to that of a pre-school child. Also, her figures had no sexuality, indicating that she was uncertain and experiencing denial about the recent sexual assault.

In her later drawings, Maryum portrayed herself in a more feminine manner by including hair and jewelry. She also drew herself larger, using more of the paper. By including recognizable arms, hands, and feet, Maryum indicated more feelings of mobility and being in control. However, the figures surrounding her continued to be somewhat incomplete, often with missing limbs or arms. Through dialogue with Maryum, the therapist learned that some of the figures with missing arms represented her male children and/or her husband and their reluctance to embrace her due to the sexual assault. Some of her figures continued to have sexual ambiguity, as evidenced by the drawing of "skirts" and other female attire over what appears to be a male figure. These are further indications of Maryum's confusion related to understanding and adjusting to the sexual assault. Maryum continues to have art therapy sessions with Farris-Dufrene as perceived as needed by Coleman, Maryum's primary therapist.

Recommendations

Maryum's treatment goals now focus on complete reunification with her husband and sons; improving her self-esteem; following through on criminal charges filed against the perpetrator; and returning to work and her normal, day-to-day activities. Coleman is involved directly in the legal proceedings related to this case, while Farris-Dufrene continues to function as the art therapist consultant.

Summary

This case is an example of how an art therapist and psychotherapist can work together to facilitate the healing of a woman who is assaulted sexually. The treatment addressed issues of how a rape victim is perceived by husband and family members from an Islamic society. The therapists had to be sensitive to religion, sexuality, and the roles of Islamic families living in Western society.

Since Maryum was assaulted sexually by a Euro-American, her husband was concerned about how she would respond therapeutically to treatment provided by a white therapist. Consequently, the husband was instrumental in identifying and selecting the primary therapist, Coleman, an African American female. Sharing similar concerns, Coleman felt it appropriate to utilize an art therapist from a multicultural background, Farris-Dufrene, a member of the Powhatan Nation.

During development of this manuscript, legal proceedings have begun against the perpetrator. Proceedings should facilitate reunification, closure, and termination for Maryum.

Questions

1. To what extent do gender, religion, and culture impact upon the therapeutic relationship?
2. What are the physiological and psychological implications of criminal physical assault on clients?
3. How can a variety of treatment modalities (for example, art therapy) facilitate positive self-esteem?
4. What is the role of a consultant in the treatment process?
5. How would one describe the relationship among Maryum, her husband, and children?

CASE STUDY #2

Brief Historical Overview

This case involves a female Caucasian in her early 50s, divorced and working as a high school home economics teacher. She sought the services of Farris-Dufrene through a local mental health directory. The client, Patricia, has been in Jungian analysis most of her adult life. Since relocating to the Midwest from her native West Coast home, she has continued Jungian analysis through weekly telephone conversations and during vacation visits home. Patricia's analyst suggested that Patricia have therapy with a local practitioner to supplement their telephone sessions. Patricia is petite, conservatively dressed, and devoutly religious. Because of her religious convictions, she has been celibate since her divorce 15 years ago; she does not have any children. She stated that her main goals in working with an art therapist were to deal with issues of loneliness; adjustment to relocating from a lively, West Coast environment to what she describes as the dreary Midwest; and conflicts with her school principal and other colleagues.

Mental Status Evaluation

Patricia is oriented to the three spheres and has a normal affect. While she is above average in intelligence, she has difficulty expressing herself verbally. Patricia is suffering from fatigue and insomnia. Due to religious beliefs, she has been abstinent for the past 15 years, since her divorce. To satisfy her sexual urges, she masturbates frequently. Memory recall is average, and she has good concentration abilities. Patricia did not present with hallucinations, delusional thoughts, or suicidal/homicidal ideation.

Empirical Observations

Assessed Psychological Impairment. A psychological evaluation conducted by Coleman revealed that Patricia has low self-esteem and is depressed. The *Tennessee Self-concept Scale* was administered to determine Patricia's level of self-esteem. The results revealed that she was below average on personal self, physical self, and social self; average on family self; and above average on moral-ethical self.

Disability Due to Impairment. The client is mildly impaired with respect to social skills; however, she is able to function occupationally.

Diagnosis (Per the DSM-IV)

<u>Patricia</u>

Axis I—Depressive Disorder, 311. 00
   Posttraumatic Stress Disorder, 309. 81
Axis II—799. 99, Diagnosis Deferred
Axis III—Fatigue, Insomnia, Anemia
Axis IV—Psychosocial and Environmental Problems: Relocation, Long-term
Divorced Status, Lack of Sexual Fulfillment, Limited Social Interaction
   Severity: Moderate
Axis V—Current GAF: 60
   Highest GAF Past Year: 60
   Previous GAF Prior to Relocation: 80

Systems Impact

Since relocating to the Midwest, Patricia is not functioning as well in her career setting and in her social life. Relations with co-workers and new community associates have been difficult. Patricia has not established any close relationships and has no social life or activity on the weekends.

Treatment Plan

Treatment Modalities. Individual art therapy was provided only three times during a three-month period. During that time, the client was referred to Coleman for psychological testing and evaluation.

Introduction. The client stated that she had a long-term interest in art therapy because of her involvement with crafts and due to the emphasis on dream imagery in Jungian analysis. She expressed an interest in illustrating her dreams and assured the art therapist that her Jungian analyst approved of the art therapy sessions. Patricia felt that she would need therapy all of her life to cope with everyday life stressors and to understand her unconsciousness.

Initial Session. Although Patricia expressed an interest in art during the initial consultation, she spent most of the first session talking and did not "feel ready to do art." "Considerable time was spent discussing her childhood and strict religious upbringing, her naivete about sexual matters, and the fact that she masturbated to satisfy her sexual needs. Patricia expressed dissatisfaction with her supervisor and other colleagues and her regrets in relocating away from her support group of family and friends. She lost her job on the West Coast because of cutbacks and the phasing out of traditional home economics classes in some school districts. Her move to the Midwest was for economic reasons. Since she was becoming very focused on career issues, the art therapist suggested that she draw a scene from her work environment (Figure 23). The scene consisted of the layout of a work/office environment. In the lower left corner, the client drew a faculty lounge, in the center an office, and on the right side a large picture window. There were no people in the scene. Patricia mentioned that she felt trapped in work bureaucracy and boxed in.

Additional Sessions. The second session took place after Patricia spent a weekend at home visiting family and friends. Patricia was much more animated and eager to draw. She had visited her analyst and seemed a little more content with her life than during the first session. During this session, she drew a landscape scene (Figure 24). Using felt-tip pens, she drew green sloping hills. Dividing the center of a page was a river and on the right side four box-shaped houses toppling each other. There were no windows, doors, or other features on the houses, and they appeared to be falling on top of each other. At the top of the drawing were three stick figures standing in a lake. Patricia described this scene as the countryside on the left and urban life on the right. Overall, the drawing was bare, sparse, with little detail and no shading. Although Patricia appeared more satisfied with her circumstances when talking to the art therapist, her drawing looked very bleak. But since she seem satisfied with her landscape and reluctant to talk about it or analyze it, the art therapist did not probe any further.

In what turned out to be the last art therapy session, Patricia began drawing right away instead of verbalizing. She produced a picture divided in half (Figure 25). On the left side of the paper she drew trees in a park encircled by a lake, with a stick figure (client) walking on a path. The figure was featureless and very tiny. The park scene had blue, green, and brown coloring. On the right side of the paper, Patricia drew a scene of cornfields using orange felt-tip pens and a grey faceless stick figure (client) walking in the cornfield. Patricia said the left side represents weekend trips to the countryside of her previous home on the West Coast. The left side portrays the boring, flat plains of the Midwest. The paper looked like two very different people had drawn on it—a depressed person on the right, and a relatively healthy, adjusted person on the left. Upon completion of the drawing, the client informed the art therapist that she was accepting a job offer back on the West Coast that would begin the following semester. Since she would be moving to the same state as her Jungian analyst in a few months, she did not feel the necessity to continue art therapy.

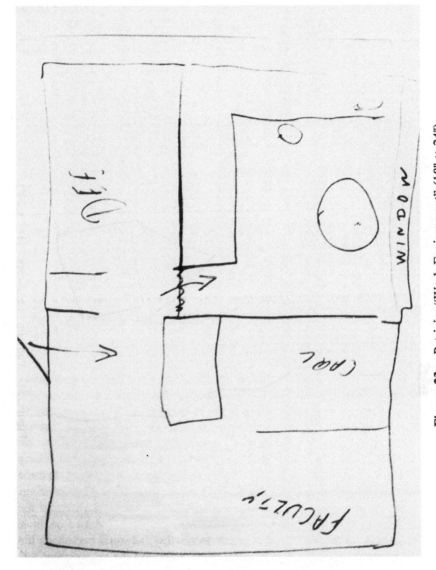

Figure 23. Patricia: "Work Environment" (18" × 24").

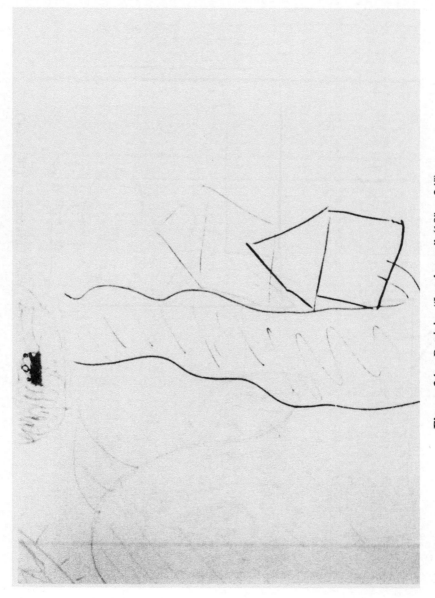

Figure 24. Patricia: "Landscape" (18" × 24").

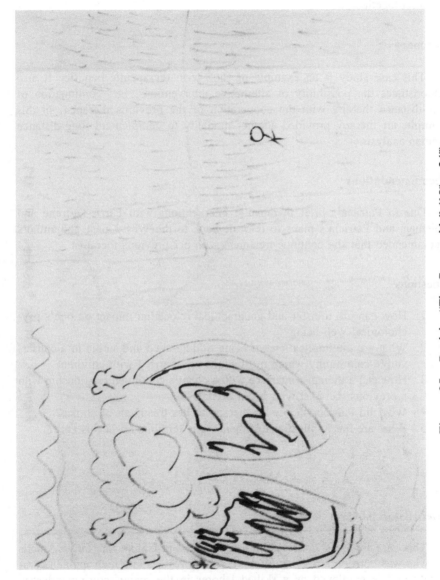

Figure 25. Patricia: "The Countryside" (18" × 24").

She thanked the art therapist for her brief intervention during the few months they met together.

Summary

This case study is an example of short-term therapeutic benefits. It also demonstrates the possibility of alternative interventions, i.e., continuation of long-distance therapy with the cooperation of the previous therapist. In this example, art therapy provided another modality to complement long-distance Jungian analysis.

Recommendations

Due to Patricia's brief therapeutic interventions with Farris-Dufrene and Coleman, and Patricia's plans to relocate back to the West Coast, the authors recommended that she continue treatment with her previous therapist.

Questions

1. How can job transfer and geographical relocation impact on one's psychological well-being?
2. What are the implications of being middle-aged and single in a conservative community where most adults are married with children?
3. How can a therapist interface with a client's continued relationship with a previous therapist who is out of state?
4. Why did Patricia choose art therapy as her treatment of choice?
5. What are the implications of therapeutic termination in this case?

CASE STUDY #3

Brief Historical Overview

This case involves James Collins, a 35-year-old Chippewa Native American who was born on a reservation but currently resides in a metropolitan community and is employed as a skilled laborer in the manufacturing industry. James initially presented to an African American female therapist for counseling due to marital issues and racial conflicts at work. Although he previously had been in treatment with a white therapist, he was somewhat anxious and apprehensive about the counseling process.

Mental Status Evaluation

The patient is oriented to the three spheres, with a broad affect. He is of average intelligence but not very verbally articulate. Although James is in counseling due to marital and job stress, he still is able to function above average in the work environment and maintains his responsibilities as a single parent.

Empirical Observations

Assessed Psychological Impairment. The therapist determined that there was no need for an extensive psychological profile in light of James' issues and concerns. Although he had not presented with major issues and concerns that would warrant this type of assessment, James also indicated vehemently that he did not subscribe to the "white man's" testing system.

Disability Due to Impairment. Because of verbal and physical altercations instigated by white coworkers, James' began to experience anxiety and lack of impulse control that led to inappropriate coping mechanisms.

Diagnosis (Per the DSM-IV)

James

Axis I—Adjustment Disorder with Depressed Mood, 309. 00
Axis II—None
Axis III—None Reported
Axis IV—Psychosocial and Environmental Problems: Work Environment, Marital Issues
    Severity: Moderate
Axis V—Current GAF: 70 (difficulty in functioning in the workplace)
    Highest GAF Past Year: 80
    Previous GAF Prior to Incident: 80

Systems Impact

The increase in racial harassment in James' work environment, coupled with his marital difficulties, began to have an adverse impact on his professional and social relationships.

Treatment Plan

Treatment Modalities. James was referred to Coleman, an African American therapist, because it was assumed that she had a more comprehensive understanding of cross-cultural issues in the workplace. James had difficulty expressing himself verbally, and he was reticent with respect to identifying his feelings. After the intake and initial assessment, Coleman decided to consult with Farris-Dufrene in order to provide a nonverbal modality and increase James' comfort level in dealing with Native American racial issues on the job.

Introduction. James had experienced several verbal and physical attacks at the workplace and consequently initiated legal proceedings against his employer. In addition to racial conflicts on the job, his estranged white wife and his former white wife were preventing the children from both of the marriages from participating in Native American activities, such as powwows and religious ceremonies. Both mothers had classified the children as white, rather than Native American, on school records and other legal documents. James was concerned that his children were losing their Indian identities and were receiving adverse information related to the Native American culture from their mothers and extended families.

The two therapists conducted extensive deliberations in order to determine the most appropriate treatment plan for James. It was decided that a combination of art therapy and psychotherapy would best facilitate James' ability to identify his feelings and develop appropriate coping mechanisms. He met with each therapist weekly on an individual basis.

Initial Session. The office environment of the Native American therapist consists of Native American art and artifacts, background Native American flute music, and burning sage for purification. Farris-Dufrene believes that this type of setting is more comfortable for clients of Indian heritage than a more traditional office environment.

Additional Sessions. James was provided with a variety of media in which he could express himself. Some of the imagery he created included scenes from his childhood living on the reservation, powwow activities, his current urban environment, and his family members. When drawing pictures of himself, his parents, or siblings, the figures were always identifiably Native American. However, his children's racial identities were ambiguous. At times, they appeared Caucasian and at other times, Native American. His pictures highlighting urban settings and his work environment included a variety of races. In drawings that included whites, their figures were large and overpowering the other racial groups portrayed. In scenes depicting his children as Caucasian, they were usually large. However, if the children were portrayed as Native American, the figures were significantly smaller. This inconsistency in size due to racial identification was broached by the therapist and led to discussion of James' feelings and attitudes about being a racial minority, both in the workplace and his wives' extended families. James acknowledged his ambivalence about his children's racial identities due to his two interracial marriages and also discussed his apprehension concerning his rationale for marriage outside of his culture on two occasions.

Through art therapy and verbal psychotherapy, James is attempting to come to terms with his low self-esteem and his inability to cope with his complex situation. This is the first time he has had a Native American role model in a professional setting. He has expressed the fact that having two minority therapists has been an inspiration for him to pursue his educational goals and objectives and, hopefully, obtain a professional position.

James is also in the process of negotiating with his estranged wife and ex-wife concerning art therapy for his five children from the two marriages. Because the children are in predominantly white school environments with all white teachers, James feels that they are lacking Native American professional role models and are not exposed to Native American and other cultures. Coleman and Farris-Dufrene use art therapy and play therapy to improve James' children's self-images in relation to cultural identity.

James has a natural inclination toward both life drawing and mechanical drafting. Consequently, art therapy was an appropriate modality for him to express his feelings. His art therapy sessions, coupled with the psychotherapy, have encouraged him to pursue courses in drafting and mechanical drawing at the community college level. The authors believe that with ongoing therapy and continuing education, James will be able to lead a more productive life and have more pride in his culture and Native American heritage. This should result in his ability to help the five children better appreciate their ethnic background.

Summary

This case illustrates the various dynamics of interracial and biracial family systems, especially in a rural, predominantly white community with a history of intolerance for racial minorities. Another significant factor is the ongoing racial harassment in the work environment, a situation in which neither the client nor therapists had the authority to mediate. This also highlights the advantages of utilizing multicultural therapists for minority clients.

Recommendations

Both therapists recommended that the client consider civil litigation against the employer. The client welcomed the suggestion; however, his attorney was not supportive in this endeavor. Mediation, unfortunately, was unsuccessful. Additional recommendations were for his children to have more contact with their Native American relatives and participate in powwows and other cultural activities. Although both therapists encouraged the two ex-wives to participate in family and individual therapy, they were uncooperative. While there were many insurmountable obstacles, the therapists are pleased with James' compliance with treatment and overall increase in self-esteem and positive racial identity.

Questions

1. What are the advantages of minority clients having the option to select minority therapists?
2. What are some of the sociological, psychological, and economic problems facing many Native Americans?
3. What are the issues encountered in interracial marriages and their impact on biracial offspring?
4. How may art therapy be beneficial to a nonverbal client?
5. In what ways can a therapist address work and stress related issues?

REFERENCE

American Psychiatric Association. (1994). *Diagnostic and statistical manual of mental disorders* (fourth edition). Washington, DC: Author.

Chapter 7

PROFESSIONAL, ETHICAL, AND LEGAL CONSIDERATIONS

The increased number of health care professionals, particularly mental health professionals, providing a variety of services has created potential legal pitfalls for the health care industry (Hopkins & Anderson, 1990). Consequently, art therapists and psychotherapists are more vulnerable to being involved in the judicial system at some time in their careers. Because of the historical experience, contemporary racial biases, and frustrations encountered by many in our society, the authors have identified specific professional, ethical, and legal issues/guidelines that they recommend should be considered/followed when providing art therapy and psychotherapeutic services. Several topics will be addressed including codes of ethics, confidentiality, civil and criminal liability, and private practice.

The American Psychological Association's *Ethical Principles of Psychologists* (American Psychological Association, 1981) is considered to be the framework for guidelines for ethical codes of behavior for the mental health profession. This code of ethics appears to be the most supported by mental health professionals from a variety of disciplines and backgrounds. It should be noted that as our industrialized, technological society continues to change, and values and mores are reconsidered, so do ethical standards and codes of behavior change. Consequently, any discussion of this topic must be within the context of contemporary issues and problems encountered by those delivering mental health services.

CODE OF ETHICS AND ETHICAL BEHAVIOR

Ethical Theory

It has been documented that ethical theory from a philosophical perspective is categorized according to descriptive ethics, metaethics, and normative ethics. *Descriptive ethics* deals with empirical evidence and observation, and from a disciplinary viewpoint has its antecedents rooted in anthropology. For example, descriptive ethics would consider the question of right versus wrong. *Metaethics* focuses on moral philosophy and is conceptual in terms of what behaviors are considered to be ethical and what the term ethical means. The resolution of specific circumstances and dilemmas is related to *normative ethics*, which would raise the question of the ethical courses of action (Margenau, 1990).

Applied ethics has emerged within the last two decades and is an attempt to explain and justify human behavior utilizing philosophical tenets. The topic of professional, ethical, and legal considerations is debated among mental health specialists as they are confronted with a myriad of issues and concerns.

Ethical Principles

Probably the assumption can be made that most mental health professionals would subscribe to the ethical principle of the value and worth of all human beings and the facilitation of human welfare. Basic ethical principles underlie the behavior of all mental health care providers and include such behaviors as educational preparation and training as it relates to professional competence, integrity, and honesty in terms of the psychotherapeutic process; and a willingness to acquire the necessary personal and professional awareness and skills to function in the global village with multicultural and diverse populations.

ETHICAL PRINCIPLES FOR ART THERAPISTS AND PSYCHOTHERAPISTS

Confidentiality and Legal Issues

The issue of confidentiality is the most fundamental concept or principle in the client-therapist relationship. While it is understood that confidentiality must be safeguarded, there are many circumstances in which this trust or communication must be broken. The landmark Tarasoff (1976) case in California is a classic illustration of the significance of confidentiality and the role and responsibility of health care providers.

Documentation

Art therapists and psychotherapists are required to maintain written and visual records of the therapeutic relationship. The purpose of these records is to document accountability, communication, and interaction between the therapist and client, and to protect citizens and the public welfare. Records should be such that those who may read them (i.e., clients, a variety of medical and other mental health professionals, insurance representatives, members of the judicial community, etc.) can capture a picture and understanding of what occurred during the therapeutic process.

Court Appearances

Art therapists and psychotherapists frequently are subpoenaed to testify in court for a variety of purposes such as child custody evaluations, alleged sexual and physical assault, and mental ability of the client to testify. Coleman has testified on several occasions concerning the aforementioned issues, and Farris-Dufrene has provided written and visual presentations to attorneys and other members of the judicial community.

Civil and Criminal Liability

Art therapists and psychotherapists may encounter an element of risk as they perform activities in the therapeutic process. Liability can be either civil or criminal and can involve court actions. The mental health professional has a responsibility to respond to civil and criminal complaints lodged by clients, consumers, other colleagues, professional associations, and the general public. For art therapists and psychotherapists to protect themselves against the possibility of civil and criminal suits, malpractice insurance policies are recommended.

PROFESSIONAL, ETHICAL, AND LEGAL CONSIDERATIONS: MULTICULTURAL AND DIVERSE POPULATIONS

For art therapists and psychotherapists working with multicultural clients, a knowledge of some of the basic elements of clients' philosophies of health and medicine may help to overcome cultural barriers between therapists and clients of different ethnic backgrounds. With respect for all cultures, art therapists and psychotherapists can better facilitate the therapeutic relationship.

Sometimes within the counseling relationship, multicultural populations may encounter barriers. Consequently, to overcome these barriers, therapists must recognize that values differ significantly from one culture to another. For example, the Eurocentric or American concept of success includes individualism, hard work, and perseverance. Many multicultural clients oftentimes do not subscribe to these Eurocentric conceptualizations of what is important in life (Coleman & Barker, 1991).

Incorporating traditional ethnic healing techniques, particularly the use of art in healing, may be extremely important. Because most minority populations are a product of both the dominant culture and their own ethnic heritage, a blend of traditional healing techniques and art therapy/psychotherapy methods may be appropriate for various social and emotional disorders.

Several factors have contributed to minority mental health concerns, including cultural breakdowns that end many of their traditional ways of life and the general disappearance of their traditional spiritual practices. Some important ethical considerations for therapists to remember when working with minority clients are the extenuating (weakening) nature of their status in American society and the less advantageous social conditions sometimes faced by these populations. Many multicultural populations must choose between two paths—the ethnic or the dominant culture path. Those who are most likely to avoid social deviance are well-grounded in both cultures. The ethical question facing therapists is how to encourage and enhance such development in both traditional/ ethnic and modern societies. Minority therapists may be better able to facilitate that development.

Some contemporary Western therapeutic techniques have similarities with traditional ethnic/indigenous healing. For example, the role of the group leader or facilitator can be compared to an elder, clan leader, or medicine person in an indigenous culture. In many cultures, group discussions are held in a circle, with each person having an opportunity to participate. Assuming that the art therapist or psychotherapist has examined his or her own value system with respect to other cultures, the use of a variety of mechanisms, including traditional techniques, may be helpful in resolving psychological concerns in the lives of clients.

Historical experiences, contemporary racial biases, and the aforementioned frustrations have motivated the authors to identify specific ethical and professional issues that they recommend should be considered when providing therapeutic services for multicultural populations.

1. Therapists should be aware of the historical, sociological, and psychological influences that prevent or inhibit minority groups from seeking mental health services.
2. Therapists should consider providing outreach activities such as workshops and seminars in order to educate minority populations concerning the efficacy of mental health services.
3. Therapists should consider the financial situations of some multicultural clients and be willing to offer services on a sliding scale and to accept Medicaid, Medicare, or other arrangements that are acceptable to both client and therapist.
4. Therapists should consider how minority populations conceptualize time and space and understand that the Eurocentric approach to punctuality may or may not be a factor when the client is seeking treatment.
5. Therapists should consider seeking and/or providing supplementary services such as day care and transportation when working with some multicultural clients.
6. Therapists should consider that multicultural and diverse populations frequently involve their family in aspects of their lives, and therefore, it may be critical to utilize a systemic approach to treatment in order to facilitate personal growth and development.

SUMMARY

Art therapists and psychotherapists have a major responsibility for understanding the professional, ethical, and legal considerations related to providing quality mental health care for clients. Each therapist must respect the value and worth of human beings, and be committed to promoting growth and development through an awareness of his or her philosophical and ethical orientation. Inevitably, therapists will, at some point in their careers, encounter civil or criminal charges based on allegations of malpractice. Consequently, art therapists and psychotherapists must be cognizant of the myriad of guidelines, rules, regulations, and legislation pertinent to their respective professions.

RECOMMENDATIONS

1. Imperatively, therapists need to have at least a general conceptualization of how the legal system functions.

2. Therapists must become familiar with all of the legal and judicial entities in their respective communities.
3. Therapists, for their protection, must carry the appropriate amount of malpractice liability insurance.
4. Therapists should have access to legal counsel.
5. Therapists must adhere to the highest ethical and professional standards of behavior.

QUESTIONS

1. In what ways do gender and race sometimes impact on legal decisions for clients?
2. What is the current legislation in your jurisdiction pertaining to physical and sexual assault?
3. What is the therapist's responsibility if physical or sexual abuse is suspected?
4. In what situations should a therapist divulge confidential information?
5. What are the possible consequences if therapists and/or clients are uninformed of their legal rights and responsibilities?

REFERENCES

American Psychological Association. (1981). *Ethical principles of psychologists.* Washington, DC: Author.

Coleman, V.D., & Barker, S.A. (1991). Barriers to the career development of multicultural populations. *Educational and Vocational Guidance, 52,* 25–29.

Hopkins, B.R., & Anderson, B.S. (1990). *The counselor and law.* Alexandria, VA: American Association for Counseling and Development.

Margenau, E.A. (Ed.). (1990). *The encyclopedic handbook of private practice.* New York: Gardner Press.

Tarasoff v. Regents of University of California, 131 Rptr. 14, 551 P. 2d 334 (1976).

Chapter 8

MULTICULTURAL ISSUES IN ART THERAPY AND PSYCHOTHERAPY

Some important considerations for art therapists and psychotherapists to remember when working with multicultural and diverse populations are the extenuating nature of minority status in American society and the less advantageous social conditions faced by many in these populations.

Frequently, multicultural and diverse populations encounter barriers in art therapy and psychotherapy. Consequently, to overcome these barriers, art therapists and psychotherapists must recognize that values differ significantly from one culture to another. For example, the Eurocentric or American concept of success includes individualism, hard work, and perseverance. However, clients from different backgrounds and cultures may have difficulty fitting into this "winner" stereotype. And sometimes, these values also may be antagonistic to the values of ethnic clients' own cultures (e.g., those cultures valuing cooperation over individualism) (Coleman & Barker, 1991).

BARRIERS

Same Versus Different Color Therapist than Client

The authors have collaborated on several cases with urban Native Americans, African Americans, Hispanic Americans, and Arab Americans. Clients oftentimes have stated that it feels appropriate to have an art therapist or psychotherapist of the same or similar ethnic or racial background because the therapist is apt to have a better understanding of cross-cultural issues and concerns. Having people of color as art therapists and psychotherapists provides role models that are instrumental in facilitating self-actualization in clients. Minority therapists, because of their experiences with racism and discrimination, may have a unique understanding of the idiosyncrasies and nuances of American life.

Values

Art therapy and psychotherapy must respect the spiritual dimensions of various cultures. Specific practices are determined by individual cultural values, beliefs, mores, folkways, and customs. Western therapeutic techniques may or may not be appropriate; however, art therapists and psychotherapists must determine the efficacy of a given approach based on consultation with each individual client. Therapists should examine critically the philosophy of Eurocentric techniques, i.e., purpose of psychotherapy, role of the therapist, function of individual or group members. In so doing, the therapist will assess if there is or is not congruence with the values and beliefs of a given minority culture. When providing art therapy or psychotherapy to individuals from different cultures, it is imperative first to understand one's own values, beliefs, attitudes, and biases.

Art therapy is based on the assumption that art and therapy are important in the integration and reintegration of personality functioning. Art therapy, because of its ability to reduce anxiety and defensiveness by exploring feelings through visual processes, is a viable treatment modality for multicultural populations. An art therapist with a similar ethnic background to the client's can better understand the special problems a given "minority" experiences (Dufrene, 1988).

The development of the roles of "minorities" in art therapy, both patients and therapists, is well-documented by Joseph (1974). The use of art for creative/therapeutic purposes by Native Americans, Africans, and Asians is being researched by an African American New York based psychiatrist named Bolling. Documentary information on Third World mental health issues is being compiled by the National Alliance of Third World Art Therapists. Contemporary medicine men/women, such as the faculty of the Traditional Indian Medicine Conferences (1985-present), are recognized nationally for helping in the current revival of traditional Native American healing methods.

To prepare art therapists to be sensitive to all their client's needs, feelings, strengths, weaknesses, and cultural perspectives is very demanding. With the cultural diversity prevalent in most parts of the United States, it is particularly difficult for an aspiring professional in the helping professions always to be aware of the subtleties needed to work with clients of varying backgrounds. The lack of interest or insensitivity to other cultures affects the treatment of various racial/ethnic groups seeking art therapy or any other type of mental health counseling (Joseph, 1974).

Art therapists have a responsibility to their clients to determine, through the most appropriate and efficient observation techniques, the extent to which clients' creative productions are influenced by ethnic, tribal, religious, and other heritage factors. True, much is universal and much is common to all human-kind, but when differences do exist, different solutions for treatment must be considered.

Caught in Two Worlds

It also is difficult for art therapists of the same ethnic background as their clients to work with those who are caught in two worlds—the world of their family origin and the world of the general American society. Researchers, students, therapists, and clients from culturally mixed backgrounds may want to understand and experience both Western and non-Western approaches to health care. Farris-Dufrene, an art therapist of Native American heritage, participates in both methods of helping people—Western versions of art therapy and traditional Native American uses of the arts for healing. To bridge the gap to both satisfy Western concepts of scientific research and education and also embrace non-Western concepts of knowledge stemming from the spiritual dimension is challenging (Dufrene, 1988).

BRIDGES

For art therapists working with clients from non-Western backgrounds, a knowledge of some of the basic elements in clients' respective philosophies of health and medicine may help to overcome cultural barriers between the art therapist and the client. With mutual respect for all cultures, art therapists and clients from varying ethnic backgrounds can facilitate a therapeutic relationship (Dufrene & Coleman, 1992).

Shamanism

Since most people of color in the United States are a product of both the dominant U.S. culture and their own family heritages, a blend of traditional healing techniques and art therapy and psychotherapy methods may be the best treatment. Almost all of the healing disciplines came originally from religious beliefs and the spiritual leaders' practices. The severance of medicine and psychology from religion has been only a recent event in the history of the world as we know it today (Tedlock & Tedlock, 1975).

Shamanic knowledge is remarkably consistent across the planet. In spite of cultural diversity and the migration and diffusion of peoples across the earth, the basic themes related to the art and practice of *shamanism* form a coherent complex. Cultural variations do exist, and yet when examining the field, there are superficial features as well as deeper structures that appear to be constant (Halifax, 1981). Trance, dance, painted drums, and shields were central to early shamanism, as they are to the continuing practice of this art today. For the shaman, the cosmos is personalized. Rocks, plants, trees, bodies of water, and two- and four-legged creatures all are animate. The world of the human being and the world of nature and spirit are essentially reflections of each other in the shaman's view of the cosmos. This special and sacred awareness of the universe is codified in song and chant, poetry and tale, carving, and painting (Dufrene, 1988).

Symbolism

The use of animals and other symbols to portray religious longings, visions, tribal affiliations, and other deep-seated beliefs is a universal phenomenon. Jung was one of the first Western therapists to show that *symbolism* produced by his patients and the symbolism found in mythologies from various parts of the world have basic similarities. The writings of Jung and Freud, based on their research in African and Asian cultures, explained the phenomena of symbolism in art dreams.

Symbols express and represent meaning. Meaning helps provide purpose and understanding in the lives of human beings. Ways of expressing and representing meaning include the symbol systems of mathematics, spoken and written language, and the arts.

One of the main functions traditional healing shares with mythology in general is the construction of a symbolic world in which the individual can feel comfortable, safe, and familiar. Sometimes this is done with mandalas. Mandala is the Sanskrit word for circle. The *mandala* is primarily an imago mundi (an idealized image of self or others); it represents the cosmos in miniature and, at the same time, the pantheon (all of the deities of a people). In a mandala, these images of world order are in the form of a schematic diagram showing the balance of forces in the symbolic universe (Sandner, 1978). Asians and Native Americans have developed this kind of mandalic form to a degree found nowhere else. They not only have drawn the mandala in sand paintings, on war shields, and in rock paintings, but also have projected it into images of space and time.

ART AS A VEHICLE

Art therapists, psychotherapists, and other mental health professionals are discovering that even the near miracles of modern Western medicine are not always adequate in themselves at solving completely all the problems of those who are ill or who wish to avoid illness. Increasingly, art therapists, psychotherapists, and other mental health professionals are seeking supplementary healing methods, and many also are engaged in personal experimentation to discover workable alternative approaches to achieving well-being. Ancient methods such as the work of shamans and other traditional healing techniques are already time-tested; in fact, they have been tested immeasurably longer, for example, than psychoanalysis and a variety of other psychotherapeutic techniques.

In contemporary American society there is a tendency to regard health and health care services as a private matter between practitioners and patients. However, health care has another meaning as a component of culture and cultural identity. This component is visible in a cross-cultural revitalization of health care that may be a key to solving the pressing health problems of multicultural American populations.

A major similarity between art therapy and traditional, indigenous healing is the recognition of the tremendous power of the healing process. When art reaches its highest levels of potential, art establishes within the confines of its symbolic world states of harmony between antagonistic forces. According to art therapist Landgarten (1981), the serious quality of clients' art hinges on the purposeful making of symbols. Disturbances of the capacity to make useful personal symbols in art can be a serious indication of pathology (Landgarten, 1981).

All over the world indigenous peoples regard art as an element of a larger activity, as part of life, and not as a separate aesthetic ideal. In most indigenous societies, the arts are aspects of public life that bring together dancing, poetry, and the plastic (two-dimensional) and graphic arts into a single function: ritual as the all-embracing expression. Art is indispensable to ritual. For example, among Native American cultures, ritual is the indigenous concept of the whole life process. Native Americans see painting as indistinct from worship and worship as indistinct from living (Highwater, 1976).

Art is highly valued for its magical power, and there is a mystical basis for aesthetic judgment among Native Americans. If the art is well made, it is "good spirit" rather than "beautiful" (Highwater, 1976).

While both art therapy and indigenous healing use the arts for healing purposes, art therapy is definitely secular in its use of the arts, while multicultural, indigenous populations do not separate art from religion. Most contemporary books on psychology, art therapy, and behaviorism leave out the spiritual component of the human mind. Some would consider it unethical and/or illegal to introduce concepts of religion/spirituality into the art therapy process in publicly funded institutions.

Despite many glaring differences between the concepts of art therapy and indigenous uses of the arts for healing, there is a recent development toward merging the disciplines. Practitioners of therapy, like practitioners of other forms of Western psychotherapy and medicine, are seeking alternative health measures from multicultural societies (Jilek, 1982).

However, in order to understand and use the arts and healing from various cultures now represented in the United States, art therapists must research ways that the arts function in non-Western societies such as African, Oceanic, Native American, and Asian. As a way of understanding art outside of one's own culture, art historian Rubin (1989) offered three relatively universal areas that delineate the ways art functions in a society. The first broad area is the establishment and proclamation of individual and group identity; the second, a didactic system that links generations in shared beliefs and behaviors; and the third, a form of technology by which people relate to their environment and secure their survival. According to this theory, all art has three properties: material (wood, ivory, clay, jade, etc.), motif (representational figures or abstract forms), and workmanship (the degree of capability the artist brings to the execution).

Viewed as such, art is not art for art's sake. Functions are implied. Due attention is given to the *purposes* of art, ranging from concrete (healing, influencing the environment) to more abstract (unifying the community, enculturation, and individual identity) (Rubin, 1989).

Rubin (1989) suggested the following types of questions to comprehend art outside of one's culture: Where does it originate? With what ethnic group does the artist identify? What people in the society use it (actually and symbolically)?

In Rubin's (1989) book, *Art as Technology: The Arts of Africa, Oceania, Native America, and Southern California*, he searched for rules and principles associated with the arts in all human societies. One of the universal factors appears to be the exploitation of both ephemeral and enduring materials. In many societies, enduring materials such as skeletal remains, crystals, sea shells, and cast metal are chosen for intrinsic symbolic content. Body art, often ephemeral, is connected with conceptions of individual identity and group membership.

Also found throughout the world are containers associated with women's art activities such as basketry and pottery. Consistently found on containers throughout the world is geometric nonrepresentational ornamentation. The designs have cultural content and philosophical meaning associated with centering, dynamic balance of complicated elements within the design field, and a striving to harmonize the natural world. The designs are representations of spirit principles or shamanic helpers and are used to solve the problem of representing spiritual entities in art (Dufrene, 1991).

In *Art as Technology* (Rubin, 1989), the author also discussed the phenomena of cultural confluence or artistic blending from diverse cultures due to encounter, discovery, or conquest. Contemporary Hispanic/Latino culture in California is a blend of indigenous Mexican Indians and their Spanish conquerors. The Hispanic "Day of the Dead" rituals are reminiscent of indigenous Mexican rituals. Mexican murals interpret Pre-Columbian, Colonial, and Modern phases of life. Symbols and motifs from diverse sources are used to interpret traditional, historical, and present events, thus creating a contemporary collective identity that unifies the Hispanic/Latino population (Dufrene, 1991).

It is useful for art therapists and psychotherapists to study the art of many cultures, especially the cultures of their respective clients. Art directs the heart of a community's values and reveals how the community functions. The arts help us understand values, beliefs, and behavioral conventions within a community (Dufrene, 1991).

PHYSICAL AND MENTAL HEALTH RELATIONSHIP

While the lack of modern technology may have forced "primitive" peoples to develop their latent shamanic powers for healing, even today it is increasingly recognized that health and healing sometimes require more than modern Western technological methods. There is a new awareness that physical and mental health are closely related—that emotional factors can play an important role in the onset, progress, and cure of illness.

A current example of a mutually supportive combination of shamanism, art therapy, and Western medicine is the work of Simonton and Matthews-Simonton in treating cancer patients. Patients use visualization techniques that resemble shamanic journeys involving inner guides that may take the physical form of a human being or an animal. Patients visualize and make drawings of their cancers, which often resemble snakes and other monsters/creatures. Simonton and Matthews-Simonton's patients often are surprised at their success in gaining relief from pain and in achieving the remission of their cancerous conditions (Harner, 1982).

SUMMARY

Comparative studies of art therapy, indigenous uses of the arts for healing, and contemporary art in multicultural/cross-cultural populations are important for art therapists working with diverse populations. Western and/or mainstream American populations also can be considered for modified uses of indigenous art and healing techniques.

RECOMMENDATIONS

Because of historical experiences of oppression and contemporary racial biases impacting on United States "people of color," Farris-Dufrene, an art therapist of Native American heritage (Powhatan), and Coleman, a Black American psychologist, have developed recommendations and guidelines for therapists working with clients from various racial/ethnic backgrounds.

1. Therapists working with diverse racial/ethnic populations should have an understanding of the cultural beliefs of the populations they serve.
2. Therapists should consider incorporating multicultural therapeutic techniques in their clinical practices.

3. Therapists should become more involved with the social issues that affect clients and place more emphasis on helping clients develop positive strengths for utilization in bringing about social change. For example, art can be used as a cohesive force with the power to bring oppressed people together, inspiring them to action.

4. People of historically oppressed, multicultural populations should be encouraged to enter mental health professions, thereby providing appropriate responses to culture-specific emotional disorders.

5. Therapists should consider the spiritual dimension of clients during evaluation and treatment. This is necessary because many multicultural populations incorporate spirituality into their healing beliefs.

6. It is recommended that more dialogue/exchange take place between Western therapists and traditional healers from various cultures.

7. It is recommended that college educators be more flexible in their requirements for adherences to the "scientific method" when research is conducted on topics that do not conform to the scientific model, i.e., shamanism or traditional healing.

8. It is recommended that the National Indian Health Board and the National Indian Health Service seek matching grants for exchange programs involving traditional Indian healers and art therapists or other health professional/educators. This recommendation also could be applicable to health organizations responsible for other ethnic constituencies such as the Association of Black Psychologists and the National Association of Black Social Workers.

9. Therapists need to be aware of their own cultural biases when working cross-culturally. When providing therapy to individuals from different cultures, it is imperative first to understand one's own values, beliefs, attitudes, and biases.

QUESTIONS

1. How have racism and oppression in the United States affected the mental health professions?

2. How do some multicultural groups perceive the concept of therapeutic services?

3. How can therapists use traditional and/or indigenous healing techniques in treatment?

4. What are the advantages of clients and therapists having similar ethnic backgrounds?

5. How have the arts traditionally been used for healing in diverse cultures?

REFERENCES

Coleman, V.D., & Barker, S.A. (1991). Barriers to the career development of multicultural populations. *Educational and Vocational Guidance, 52,* 25–29.

Dufrene, P., & Coleman, V. (1992). Counseling Native Americans: Guidelines for group process. *The Journal for Specialists in Group Work, 17,* 229–234.

Dufrene, P. (1991). Art as technology: The arts of Africa, Oceania, Native America, and Southern California. *Art Therapy, 8,* 29–31.

Dufrene, P. (1988). *A comparison of the traditional education of Native American healers with the education of American art therapists.* Ann Arbor, MI: University Microfilms International.

Halifax, J. (1981). *The shaman.* New York: Crossroad.

Harner, M. (1982). *The way of the shaman.* New York: Bantam Books.

Highwater, J. (1976). *Songs from the earth: American Indian painting.* Boston, MA: Little, Brown & Company.

Jilek, W. (1982). *Indian healing: Shamanic ceremonialism in the Pacific Northwest.* Surrey, British Columbia, Canada: Hancock House.

Joseph, C. (1974). *Art therapy and the third world.* New York: Cliff Publishers.

Landgarten, H. (1981). *Clinical art therapy.* New York: Brunner/Mazel.

Rubin, A. (1989). *Art as technology: The arts of Africa, Oceania, Native America, and Southern California.* Beverly Hills, CA: Hillcrest Press.

Sandner, D. (1978). *Navaho symbols of healing.* New York: Harcourt, Brace & Javonavich.

Tedlock, D., & Tedlock, B. (1975). *Teachings from the American earth: Indian religion and philosophy.* New York: Liveright.

Chapter 9

CAREER DEVELOPMENT ISSUES IN ART THERAPY AND PSYCHOTHERAPY

The career development of America's varied population is an important topic in contemporary mental health. Consequently, the career development of art therapists and psychotherapists is gaining significance as the need for health care providers increases. Coleman (1989) has designed a Model of Career Development, and Coleman and Barker (1992) have designed a Model of Career Development for a Multicultural Workforce. Both these models have applications for art therapists, psychotherapists, and other mental health professionals. The Model of Career Development will be discussed in detail in this chapter.

HISTORICAL DEVELOPMENT

Organized attempts for art therapists to form a cohesive professional group began in 1969 with the founding of the American Art Therapy Association (AATA). There are now a number of state and regional art therapy associations. The development of art therapy literature devoted to theory building and research, gradual until the 1960s, has been proceeding more rapidly in the past decade. *The American Journal of Art Therapy*, founded by the late Elinor Ulman in 1961, was for a long time the only professional journal in the field. In 1983, AATA began publishing a new journal, *Art Therapy*. The American Art Therapy Association also developed registration procedures for art therapists who have worked a certain number of years, completed extensive study, and published. This registration is designated ATR (Art Therapist Registered). Plans are now underway to develop a national license/certification for art therapists.

In 1969, the first two graduate programs leading to a master's degree in art therapy were announced. Presently, there are approximately 50 programs offering training in art therapy. The American Art Therapy Association has designated the master's degree as constituting the professional entry level. The organization has developed mechanisms for the endorsement of training programs offered by clinical facilities, as well as programs leading to academic degrees.

Prior to the 1990s, art therapists usually worked in educational or clinical settings under somewhat limited constraints. In institutions of higher learning, such as universities or psychoanalytic institutes, art therapy educators taught/teach art therapy skills to potential art therapists, art teachers with special education students mainstreamed in their classes, psychologists, social workers, psychiatrists, and other mental health professionals seeking alternative therapy techniques. In clinical settings, such as hospitals and mental health clinics, art therapists were/are part of a therapeutic team that diagnoses and treats emotionally disturbed individuals. In schools, especially special education schools, art as therapy is stressed by art therapists/educators (Dufrene, 1988).

However, in the 1990s, art therapy has grown and developed to reach new populations in new settings. Art therapy has expanded beyond its initial applications in psychiatric clinical settings and special education classes to now include battered women in shelters, incest victims, international refugees, clients with various physiological disorders and/or psychological disorders, and victims of posttraumatic stress syndrome (Wadeson, 1989).

The broadening of art therapy into diverse institutional settings is partly a reflection of society's changing needs in the areas of social services. Careers in art therapy now encompass a variety of work sites and populations. Working with different populations requires training in specialized fields, particularly when working with clients who have physiological problems or when treating clients from cultures other than those of the art therapists.

The Model of Career Development (Coleman, 1989), with applications for art therapists and psychotherapists, identifies issues that are relevant to art therapists and psychotherapists as they examine their own career issues. The Model of Career Development (Coleman, 1989) has its antecedents in the theoretical frame of Super's (1957) Development Self-Concept Theory of Vocational Behavior. Super has suggested that individuals attempt to implement their self-concept by choosing to enter the occupation they perceive as providing the most opportunity for self-expression. He also indicated that the specific behaviors that individuals engage in are a function of their stage of life development. The Model of Career Development for a Multicultural Workforce (Coleman & Barker, 1992) also emphasizes self-assessment, which includes an identification of one's values, interests, abilities, and personality. According to the Model of Career Development for a Multicultural Workforce, these four areas comprise the core of knowledge necessary for career exploration for art therapists and psychotherapists.

Self-concept Development

Super, Starishevsky, Matlin, and Jordaan (1963) examined self-concept theory as it pertained to vocational development. They described self-concept development as being comprised of the processes of formation, translation, and implementation of self-concepts.

Self-esteem

Self-esteem, or self-acceptance, is a dimension of self-concepts (Super et al., 1963). Self-esteem is the feeling tone or how one feels about oneself. Persons with high levels of self-esteem feel a sense of value and worth, like themselves, have confidence in themselves, and act accordingly. Those with low levels of self-esteem are doubtful about their own worth; see themselves as undesirable; often feel anxious, depressed, and unhappy; and have little faith or confidence in themselves. Feelings of high or low self-esteem, of course, affect the planning for, entering, adjusting to, progressing in, and leaving of occupational endeavors or other life experiences.

MODEL OF CAREER DEVELOPMENT

The Model (Coleman, 1989) consists of six components: (1) Introduction and Orientation; (2) Self-assessment; (3) Decision Making; (4) Educational, Occupational, and Community Information; (5) Preparation for Work, Leisure, and Retirement; and (6) Research and Evaluation.

Introduction and Orientation

The purpose of this component is to introduce the concept and process of career development, and to provide a working definition. Career development is defined as an ongoing, lifelong process, beginning at birth and continuing throughout life. This component focuses on the acquisition of information and skills about self and the world of work. Career development is different from the traditional definition of career education/vocational guidance in that the goal of career development is to facilitate the self-actualization of the individual, rather than to respond to labor market demands.

Self-assessment

This component, considered the foundation of the career development process (Coleman, 1989), focuses on four variables: values, interests, abilities, and personality as they related to career development. *Values* are significant in that when one chooses a career, one is choosing a value system and a lifestyle. Not only are *vocational interests* explored, but also *avocational interests*—what does one like to do for fun? *Abilities,* achievements, and accomplishments are important, along with the type of *personality* the individual possesses.

Academic assessment with respect to intelligence, learning styles, academic deficiencies, and cultural influences is determined in relationship to the aforementioned personal factors. From the academic and personal information, an individual learning plan is designed and correlated with career aspirations.

All of this information should assist an individual in responding appropriately to the question, "Who Am I?" Coleman (1989) held self-assessment to be the most critical element in the career development process.

Decision Making

Decision making is also a critical component and is a skill that can be learned. Principles, strategies, and styles are explored, with particular emphasis being placed on the individual's strategies and styles of decision making. It is important to underscore that all individuals utilize all of the various strategies and styles, and one strategy or style is not better than another. Any given strategy or style may afford one the opportunity to make positive, satisfying, and appropriate decisions. For example, individuals may utilize one strategy for career decisions, another strategy for decisions related to the family, and yet a third for decisions involving friends.

Educational, Occupational and Community Information

This component identifies the occupational opportunities for the 1990s and twenty-first century, and includes the educational requirements to pursue those opportunities. Resources such as educational institutions, business and industry, fraternal and professional organizations, alumni, and community agencies provide important contributions to the career development process. The educational training and professional development of art therapists and psychotherapists is changing in the technological world. How information and resources are utilized will have a significant impact on the ability of this population to achieve its career goals and aspirations.

Preparation for Work, Leisure, and Retirement

This component focuses on the "nuts and bolts" of the job search such as resume preparation, interviewing, and job maintenance skills. Because leisure is prominent and important in one's life, a discussion of the importance of recreational activities is included. And with the increased average life span, retirement assumes a different role in one's life than it did in the past. It is apparent that one should prepare for these later years.

Art therapists and psychotherapists must understand that they have a variety of sustainable skills and talents that are transferable to a myriad of career opportunities.

Research and Evaluation

Research and evaluation are an essential component of the career development model. Issues to be explored and researched include, but are not limited to, the self-esteem, vocational maturity, and decision making of art therapists and psychotherapists.

SUMMARY

Art therapists and psychotherapists are facing a multitude of challenges as health care reform, particularly mental health care, undergoes massive changes. The success of these mental health professionals will depend upon their activities related to the career development process. The model described in this chapter can be utilized as a tool for the in-depth self-assessment and analysis of art therapists and psychotherapists in order to determine their roles in our multicultural, global village. Art therapists and psychotherapists possess the knowledge, skills, and talents to influence mental health policy at the municipal, state, regional, national, and international levels. In the 1990s and twenty-first century, art therapists and psychotherapists must adapt a variety of roles and functions and assume active responsibility for the success of the equitable delivery of mental health services to clients.

RECOMMENDATIONS

1. In order to increase the numbers of mental health professionals from multicultural and diverse backgrounds, it is necessary to provide scholarships and other financial assistance when needed.
2. Mental health careers must be presented to adolescents as viable career options when considering post-secondary education.
3. Higher education courses and programs in mental health should include a discussion of the variety of career options.
4. Mental health professionals must examine carefully their values, interests, abilities, and personality as these pertain to career development goals and objectives.
5. Professionals in mental health must have ongoing training and continuing education in order to keep abreast of new developments in mental health fields.

QUESTIONS

1. What do you consider to be the career development opportunities for mental health professionals in the twenty-first century?
2. How do you feel health reform will impact the role of the mental health provider?
3. What type of training do you think will be necessary for mental health professionals in the future?
4. What is the relationship between licensing and health insurance reimbursement?
5. As the population in the United States becomes more diverse, how will that impact the career development of mental health professionals?

REFERENCES

Coleman, V.D. (1989). *A model of career development*. Unpublished manuscript. West Lafayette, IN: Purdue University.

Coleman, V.D., & Barker, S.A. (1992). A model of career development for a multicultural workforce. *International Journal for the Advancement of Counseling, 15,* 187-195.

Dufrene, P. (1988). *A comparison of the traditional education of Native American healers with the education of American art therapists.* Ann Arbor, MI: University Microfilms International.

Super, D.E. (1957). *The psychology of careers.* New York: Harper & Row.

Super, D.E., Starishevsky, R., Matlin, N., & Jordaan, J.P. (1963). *Career development: Self-concept theory.* New York: College Entrance Examination Board.

Wadeson, H. (Ed.). (1989). *Advances in art therapy.* New York: John Wiley & Sons.

Chapter 10

IMPLICATIONS FOR MENTAL HEALTH PROFESSIONALS

The development of psychoanalysis in the United States during the early part of the twentieth century laid fertile ground for the future discipline of art therapy. Because of psychoanalysis' ability to contact the unconscious and its inner imagery through dream analysis, imagery later manifested itself visually through art therapy. Freud and Jung's beliefs that dream symbolism had meaning and provided messages from the unconscious began the conceptual reasoning for art therapy (Junge, 1994).

In the United States, intellectuals and artists became intrigued with psychoanalysis and its emphasis on free association. Naumburg, considered the mother of art therapy, became involved in analysis and used some of its principles in developing her art therapy theories that were used in the school she founded—the Walden School in New York—and in her private practice (Junge, 1994).

American's attitudes toward mental health changed in the latter part of the twentieth century. As mental illness became less stigmatized, more Americans opted for treatment privately and in hospitals. Art therapists were hired to work in psychiatric hospitals as part of therapeutic teams. During the 1950s, the development of outpatient clinics allowed more people to receive mental health services, and art therapists also became involved in that therapeutic milieu. With the advent of group and family therapy in the 1950s and 1960s, art therapists and other mental health providers reached an even wider audience. Contact with other clinicians and the establishment of graduate art therapy programs in the 1960s and 1970s increased art therapy's visibility and working alliances with various other types of psychotherapy.

The goals of art therapy and psychotherapy are more encompassing than those of recreation or education. Art therapy attempts to reach people with numerous problems through art and to fulfill the human need for self-expression in a society that is becoming increasingly mechanized. Art therapy is a vehicle for awakening dormant creativity, and psychotherapy assists people in verbalizing their unspoken and unresolved conflicts. Together, art therapy and psychotherapy contribute to restoring the cognitive/intellectual, emotional/affect, and creative/inspiration vacuums in today's stress-driven, technological, impersonal, and often unsafe world.

Art therapy and psychotherapy can lead clients of all ages to better understandings of their unconscious through dream interpretation, both verbally and visually. Both therapies help in the investigation of developmental phases and of psychic structure, and in the study of the ego (Kramer, 1993). Art therapists are cognizant of the relationship between graphic form and character structure. With the advent of psychoanalytic ego psychology, art therapists were able to better recognize that inner consistency and unity of form and content in art were the work of the ego and became more attentive to the aesthetic qualities of their clients' artwork (Kramer, 1993).

For various reasons, many art therapists hesitate to concern themselves with the artistic quality of their clients' art products. The tenet, applicable to both art therapy and psychotherapy, of accepting all products, regardless of content and form, seems contradictory to assessing aesthetic quality. Additionally, art therapists have to find a balance between art and therapy. Whereas the field of therapy and mental health are on an upward trend, the worth of the field of art is in a state of flux and under constant scrutiny by the media and conservative politicians. Kramer (1993) speculated on the future of art/art therapy:

> It is not surprising that art therapists have been inclined to stay close to the more promising field of psychotherapy. Ultimately, however, these very conditions force the art therapist to focus upon the *art* in art therapy. There is, in our opinion, evidence that the lack of active art experiences and the concomitant saturation with pseudo-art among large segments of the population constitute a pathogenic condition. The art therapist is in a position both to contribute to the understanding of this condition and to help develop methods of dealing with it. As concern over the function of the total environment in the understanding of emotional difficulties becomes more widespread, art therapy will join forces with the new field of community psy-

chiatry, which focuses on the relationship between sociocultural conditions and the epidemic rise of specific syndromes of emotional disturbance. (p. 6)

FLEXIBILITY OF COLEADERSHIP

In collaborating together on many cases, and when working individually as therapists, the authors approached art therapy and psychotherapy in myriad ways, depending on their clients' needs. In some situations, art therapy was practiced as a specialized form of psychotherapy, and at other times, art therapy functioned utilizing the creative process of art as the main therapeutic agent. In cases where art was the key factor, healing and recovery were dependent on the psychological dynamics that occur during the creative process.

In working with clients who used Coleman as the primary therapist, Farris-Dufrene's art therapy skills were used on an adjunctive and/or consultative basis. Visual imagery served to complement and/or replace the verbal exchanges between Coleman and her patients. At times, with deeply disturbed, homicidal, and/or suicidal patients, both therapists consulted a psychiatrist for further clinical supervision.

ART THERAPY AS PREPARATION
FOR PSYCHOTHERAPY

In the majority of the authors' clinical situations, especially when working with families, children were more receptive to art therapy than adult clients who preferred an intellectual, verbal approach. In general, children enjoy art. Children in elementary school, during the latency and preadolescent stages (approximately 6 through 12 years old), are especially accessible to the emotionally rewarding aspects of engaging in art activities. Even children with a wide variety of diagnosed disturbances can engage themselves in the creative process. Kramer (1993) observed art therapy's potential effect on children:

> The confrontation that creative work induces resembles the confrontation in psychoanalysis and in psychoanalytically oriented psychotherapy in certain respects. The amorphous condition of the art material and the lack of specific directions for forming it are analogous to the blank quality of the therapeutic relationship. This freedom induces the child to form the art material or the relationship in his

> own image. In both situations, the child is confronted in the course
> of time with many aspects of himself. He learns to know who he is,
> how he feels, and what he can do. However, there are differences.
> (p. 32)

In verbally oriented psychotherapy, the relationship between the child and the therapist is the main factor in the therapeutic relationship. The dynamics between the two people are the primary tools whether the child is talking to the therapist, playing with toys, or remaining quiet. The constancy is the presence of the psychotherapist.

However, making art involves the child in the invention of his or her own world and is an egocentric process. The art product, whether it is a self-portrait, a family sculpture, or a drawing of the client's house, contains parts of the child's self-identity. At times, aspects of that self that are portrayed visually may cause a confrontation with oneself. The child's pathology may become more self-evident. Failures and conflicts may arise during the creative process. If handled appropriately by the art therapist, the self-confrontations, failures, and risk taking that occur while making art can bring about personality changes in the child. Visual expression of traumatic events can help children temporarily cope with the negative experiences in their lives. However, art therapy by itself usually does not resolve profound emotional disturbance (Kramer, 1993).

For many clients, children and adults, art therapy and psychotherapy can complement and reinforce each other. Art therapy can facilitate and prepare the client for the symbolic interchanges that occur in various types of psychotherapy. Clients being treated by a psychotherapist become more aware of themselves and in turn create art that contains more personal meaning and emotional impact; thus, art offers an arena for replaying the inner conflicts and changes that occur while undergoing psychotherapy treatment (Kramer, 1993).

ACCOUNTABILITY OF COLEADERSHIP

Cotherapy (e.g., art therapy and psychotherapy) sets up a system of accountability. A phenomenon that often precipitates inner conflicts and changes in the therapist-client relationship is transference/countertransference, i.e., the tendency to transfer emotions from past experiences onto people (in this case onto the therapist) who become important to one in later life. Therapy induces the transference of feelings, fears, wishes, and fantasies onto the therapist. Effective psychotherapists remain receptive to their clients communications and respond in a manner that is empathetic. Sometimes even the most knowledgeable therapist may experience vulnerability from their patients' reactions/transference and react inappropriately because of unresolved issues in the therapist's past. In those situations, countertransference can impede the therapeutic process. Even though transference may not manifest as an important issue in adjunctive and/or consultative art therapy, art therapists must be aware of the possibility. Working as a team, the authors are available to provide feedback to one another if and when transference/countertransference does occur.

SUMMARY

The authors feel that the cases shared with readers (colleagues, students, lay persons) relay the power of art therapy and psychotherapy to bring about lasting, positive changes in peoples' lives. In their work with children, the authors have witnessed art's capacity to relieve stress, pressures, and tensions, often channeling negative aggression into constructive energy. For many clients, children and adults, art therapy has offered temporary relief for their continual struggle in dysfunctional, often abusive families. Unfortunately, for some clients, therapeutic intervention proved insufficient to relieve problems caused by overwhelming external, societal factors such as racial, gender, and class oppression; extreme poverty; and a hostile societal environment. But as therapists from multicultural backgrounds, the authors are sensitive to societal issues and committed to political activism that will enable clients of all ethnicities to reap the benefits of therapy—benefits that can, under the right conditions, effect positive changes in their personalities.

Today, many areas of the United States (urban and rural) are in economic despair. Increasingly, mental health professionals are faced with insurance cutbacks, mental health budget slashing, and a managed care mental health philosophy that focuses on the etiology of biological determinism in mental illness and attempts to discount psychotherapy (Junge, 1994). During economic crises, therapists may feel threatened about their career potential and attempt to align themselves with more "respected" disciplines, forging relationships with more so-called "reputable" accrediting organizations. Art therapists may seek alliances with psychotherapists/psychologists, and in turn psychologists/psychotherapists will try to unite with psychiatrists and other medical doctors. Although these unions may be pragmatic economically, the authors feel that art therapists and psychotherapists must always retain their unique, individual qualities of freedom, creativity, inventiveness, and commitment to healing, regardless of external factors that attempt to threaten the essence of their respective disciplines.

But despite the aforementioned challenges for both art therapists and psychotherapists, the authors are optimistic about their work with clients of all ages. The authors are confident that the blending of two fields, which respect both the creative and psychological processes, can allow individuals with diverse backgrounds and disorders to symbolically and positively experiment with ideas and feelings; to sort out life's complexities, contradictions, and often unfairness; to transcend internal/external conflicts; and most of all, to have the capacity to love and be loved.

RECOMMENDATIONS

It should be apparent that the blending of art therapy and psychotherapy is an appropriate orientation for mental health professionals. Specific recommendations for applications of "blending" related to counseling, training, research, program development, and policy are discussed below.

Counseling

It seems apparent that art therapy and psychotherapy are a viable modality for working with children, adolescents, and adults. The various techniques used in art therapy and psychotherapy allow the client to interpret experiences that will enhance his or her understanding of the self.

Training

There is a need for post-secondary institutions to educate mental health professionals to provide a more diverse spectrum of treatment modalities. Courses in anthropology, history, sociology, and political science should be mandatory requirements in graduate programs in counseling and related disciplines. The recruitment and retention of multicultural populations into art therapy and psychotherapy programs will help alleviate some of the racism and discrimination that some clients encounter in therapeutic situations.

Research

Most research conducted in art therapy and psychotherapy has been investigated by researchers of the dominant culture. Much of this research is debatable with respect to the methodology and its generalizability across cultures. As more individuals from multicultural populations acquire advanced degrees, this situation should be ameliorated.

Program Development

Programs utilizing art therapy and psychotherapy can have a significant impact on the personal growth and development of clients. Program development coupled with the design of instructional materials related to art therapy and psychotherapy can provide tools for addressing the issues, needs, and concerns of those seeking mental health services.

Policy

Advocacy for the human rights of clients is a role that art therapists and psychotherapists must assume. Policies should be considered that would facilitate the self-awareness of all individuals in the 1990s and twenty-first century.

REFERENCES

Junge, M. (1994). Politics and poetics: The acquired wisdom of the art therapist. *Art Therapy, 11,* 288–293.

Kramer, E. (1993). *Art therapy with children.* Chicago, IL: Magnolia Street Publishers.

INDEX

ABOUT THE AUTHORS

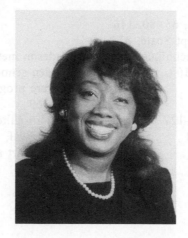

Victoria D. Coleman, Ed.D., NCC, LCSW, LMFT, is a counseling psychologist and associate professor of vocational education at Purdue University in West Lafayette, Indiana. She has a B.A. in political science and an M.A. in U.S. and Latin American history from The University of Iowa, an M.S.Ed. in counselor education from Northern Illinois University, and an Ed.D. in counseling psychology from Rutgers University. Her career spans higher education, mental health, corporate America, and social services; and she has held positions at Northwestern University, the University of Illinois, American Airlines, Educational Testing Service, the State University of New York, and the YWCA.

Dr. Coleman's research interests include the career development of multicultural and diverse populations, specifically, Black Americans, Hispanic

Americans, Native Americans, Asian-Pacific Americans, student athletes, and women. She has published extensively in these areas.

An African American female and entrepreneur, Dr. Coleman is also president/owner of The Coleman Group, a private practice and management consulting firm with offices in West Lafayette, IN, Detroit, MI, and Las Vegas, NV. She travels nationally and internationally conducting workshops for business, industry, government, educational institutions, and professional associations, and evaluates schools for accrediting.

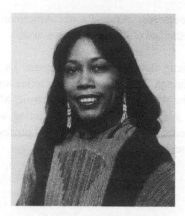

Phoebe M. Farris-Dufrene, Ph.D., A.T.R., NCC, LCSW, is an art therapist and associate professor of art and design at Purdue University in West Lafayette, Indiana. She has a B.A. in fine arts from the City University of New York, an M.P.S. in art therapy from the Pratt Institute, and a Ph.D. in art education from the University of Maryland. Dr. Farris-Dufrene, a member of the Powhatan Nation, has been a consultant for museums and galleries specializing in Native American art. She has provided expertise for mental health agencies that address the issues, needs, and concerns of Native American populations.

Dr. Farris-Dufrene has worked as an art therapist and IEP developer in special education schools in Washington, D.C. and Maryland. During that time, she also was a consultant on drug abuse prevention for the District of Columbia, a consultant for the U.S. Department of Indian Education, and a university supervisor for graduate art therapy students at George Washington University.

As an art therapist with a focus on multicultural populations, Dr. Farris-Dufrene has conducted research in Mexico (Fulbright Scholar), Cuba, and Brazil. She is active as a photographer, documenting Native American art and culture in the Eastern United States and the Caribbean. Dr. Farris-Dufrene maintains a private practice.